MW00452583

*Lessons from
the Damned*

WITHDRAW

Lessons from the Damned

....

Queers, Whores, and Junkies Respond to AIDS

Nancy E. Stoller

University of California, Santa Cruz

Routledge
New York and London

Published in 1998 by
Routledge
29 West 35th Street
New York, NY 10001

Published in Great Britain by
Routledge
11 New Fetter Lane
London EC4P 4EE

Copyright © 1998 by Routledge
Printed in the United States of America on acid free paper.

All rights reserved. No part of this book may be reprinted or repro-
duced or utilized in any form or by any electronic, mechanical or other
means, now known or hereafter invented, including photocopying and
recording or in any information storage or retrieval system, without
permission in writing from the publishers.

Library of Congress Cataloging-in-Publication Data

Stoller, Nancy E.
Lessons from the damned: queers, whores, and junkies respond to AIDS
/ Nancy Stoller.
p. cm.
Includes bibliographical references and index.
ISBN 0-415-91960-6 (hb). —ISBN 0-415-91961-4 (pb)
1. AIDS (Disease)—Social aspects—United States. 2. AIDS
(Disease)—Political aspects—United States. 3. Minorities—Health and
Hygiene—United States. 4. Social action—United States. 5. Social
movements —United States. I. Title.
RA644.A25S756 1998
362.'969792'00973—dc21   97-21462
                                                              CIP

For my mother,
Ruth Klarberg Richman,
and in memory of Nina Fortin
and Peter Canavan.

Table of Contents

Acknowledgments

Although the serious writing of this book began in 1995, the material on which the work is based began to assert itself ten years before that, in 1985. Thus, I have many people to thank. First and foremost are the many dedicated AIDS workers whose stories are told here through the organizations where they worked. They were volunteers, staff, administrators, and board members. Their occupations range from prostitution to medicine. They are the activists who have shaped the U.S. response to the epidemic. Whatever the imperfections of the community response may be, we must always remember that individually and collectively we all did the very best we could with very limited guidance.

Secondly my profound thanks to those whose words appear in quotations throughout the book. Some agreed to be interviewed. Others let me tape their talks. And in a few cases, the words you read come from public events. While the speakers knew their talks were being recorded, they were unaware that their words would end up in this book. To these, I hope I have quoted you well and fairly.

The book took initial shape with the help of my partners in The Four Tops: Allan Berube, John D'Emilio, and Estelle Freedman. Sandra Butler, Moher Downing, Luis Kemnitzer, Cheri Pies, Chris Ponticelli, Helen Vozenilek, and Doris Brin Walker read various drafts. Wendy Chapkis, David Whittier, and Christine Wong handled many research tasks. Carter Wilson, Cindy Patton, Helen Longino, Gwendolyn Shaw, and Catherine Tourette-Turgis improved the quality of my analysis in key areas. Zoe Sodja retyped and standardized the text and tables many times. I owe a special debt to my editor, Marcia Freedman, who was both reassuring and critical in perfect proportions. Haile Ben Shaw-Miller provided entertainment and distraction. Financial support has come primarily from the Regents of the University of California.

Tara, Sam Puckett, Jeff Amory, and Vito Russo died while the project developed. They were unable to check the final versions of the quotations I chose. Vito, especially, has been an inspiration to me as an activist and an intellectual. Everything I have written here, I have asked myself, what would Vito have thought about it? Sometimes I am sure he would have disagreed, but then that would have been fine, too.

List of Illustrations

Preface:
From the Grass Roots

Listening to the stories of a panel of eighteen long-term AIDS activists convened in 1994 to discuss the history of the epidemic,[1] I was struck by how multifaceted that history is and must be, not only because every individual has a unique story, but also because there are so many structural splits which sever the potential commonality of people with HIV infection. Gay men are divided by race and class, African Americans by class as well as the national and local politics of drugs and crime; some are advantaged by gender or by access to health care. And all of us are separated by our limited experience with other cultures.

The organizations represented on the panel ranged from the center of the AIDS established order to the identified margins of the movement. Their divergent cultural, social, and political values were expressed in their organizational values and strategies.

Here are some of the voices I heard that day, voices that inspired the questions and concerns that have led me to write this book.

Novella Dudley, African-American founder of Women Resourcing Women in Chicago, spoke of the rift of gender.

> I was infected in 1979, but "women didn't get this. Women didn't have HIV." So I was misdiagnosed for years. I was going from doctor to doctor. When I finally did get a diagnosis, there were no [other] women. I thought I was a freak. "I'm the only one with this virus." And what I did, I knew that the gay community in Chicago had to fight for what they got. I went to them, and I said, "I'm a woman, a Black woman, living with this virus. Can you help me meet my needs, which are different from yours?" They were very helpful. And from there on, I began to see women but they weren't being diagnosed the same way that I wasn't. They were coming into the emergency rooms with opportunistic infections or dying, because they still didn't know that they were at risk. I wanted women to stop dying and to be able to live and know about this epidemic, and not turn their heads because the media said, and our government said, that women didn't get this virus.[2]

Ron Rowell, Executive Director of the National Native American AIDS Prevention Center in Oakland, California, recalled the invisibility of Native Americans.

> I was at the first Minority AIDS Conference. There was a uniformed Public Health Service person who was not an American Indian who spoke for ten minutes on

Saturday night about AIDS and he showed some slides. One slide showed a guy in a war bonnet . . . . He concluded that AIDS was not going to be a problem in Indian country. I was sitting there with four other American Indians at that conference, one of whom was the medical director of the Navajo Nation and had five young people with AIDS for whom he was providing care at that time. I remember that we almost collapsed in tears. We were so frustrated; we had a hard time believing that this was the way things were coming down.

Following that there was a lot of fire in us. We decided that this was unacceptable. We were going to change it. We had a meeting at the CDC [Centers for Disease Control] I remember. They said that we shouldn't be considered part of the new funding for organizations of color because we had very low numbers of people infected with AIDS. What they didn't know, obviously, was that we had very high rates of sexually transmitted diseases. We had so many people who were substance abusers. A lot more intravenous drug-users than most people have. In a prevention program, that's what you have to look at. We had that to face, that too.[3]

Suki Ports, a Japanese American and founder/director of New York City's Minority AIDS Task Force, recounted her frustration with past and present racism:

In October of 1985, I was asked by the Council of Churches of the City of New York to pull together a conference. But when I called the Department of Health I was asked, "Why do you want to plan a conference on minorities and AIDS? What does that have to do with AIDS? It's only white gay men and drug addicts." So then I called the Department of Health in New York State and I said, "I'm trying to plan a conference on minorities and AIDS and I need to have somebody come and speak to the conference," and that person said, "Why would you want to talk about a minority conference on AIDS? It is only white gay men and drug addicts." . . .

It is very hard to accept the fact that we are very racist in this disease. We are very classist in this disease, and those are words that are very hard for some of us to hear without getting very defensive and saying "I'm not! She's not talking about me." Well, try it out a little because we are all sharing a very serious problem here.[4]

These voices are people of color who fought the exclusion of their communities from AIDS prevention and care. White speakers were also at the conference. Both the women and the men who spoke revealed genuine ambivalence and confusion about race, racism, and the epidemic. The desire to avoid difference is strong among white participants in the movement, who in the 1990s wish to acknowledge diversity but find it hard to challenge structural racism and sexism.

Here is Sally Fisher, the founder of the AIDS Mastery Workshop, Northern Lights Alternative, speaking at the 1994 conference.

In the beginning it was pretty much gay white people. I'm going to skip that and end about how this has switched . . . . One day in New York I was doing a workshop and we made a connection with a rehab house that had suddenly discovered they had a lot of

HIV in it. And so I walked into this room to do a workshop on a Friday night and it was like over here were a lot of gay white men all dressed up fabulous and over here were a lot of junkies and not happy. People were all slumped over and they were all looking at each other like the other guys had the plague. I thought this was going to be one of those weekends from hell. What I discovered . . . is that basically what we share is a human equation of a likeness not difference. Underneath it all we have souls and we have issues and we have lives where we have more in common than we have differences. I applaud the differences, because our differences are part of our uniqueness and what we can bring into the pot. But on the other hand, the more we look at those differences and point fingers at each other, the less consolidation and energy we have to go forward.

Signaling the "privileging," or foregrounding, of white and gay experience of the epidemic, several other white panelists at the conference also described the epidemic as originating in the gay white community. An acknowledgment of the exclusion of minority voices was heard in the comments of Michael Colbruno of the San Francisco *Bay Area Reporter*. In his phrasing, "we" means white people:

Another thing that I want to talk about with the book [*And the Band Played On*].[5] This book chronicles the AIDS epidemic, but it doesn't do a good job. It puts a lot out there. It tells a story that needed to be told, and I loved Randy a lot, but there are two things that I heard today already on this panel. "Black people didn't have AIDS" when this book was written. We know [from the panel] that's a lie. "Women didn't have AIDS" when this book was written. And we know that's a lie. And the reason is because at that time we didn't include everyone in the discussion. We didn't do things like this and we didn't put together the history that needs to be told because I've heard it said a million times if one person has AIDS, we all have AIDS. The sad reality is that's very true.

"If one person has AIDS, we all have AIDS." This bit of received wisdom originally meant that everyone in a community, a society, a world is affected, even if most are HIV-negative. Here, Colbruno confounds that meaning with the complaint by members of minority communities that the rates of infection are higher among them and that the virus has been there just as long as in these other locations.

When the Centers for Disease Control's director of AIDS programs, James Curran, spoke of the early days of the epidemic, he also remembered gay people at the center. His words unintentionally demonstrated his estrangement from poor African-American and Latino communities.

CDC was then doing what it does best, responding rapidly, doing epidemiological assessments and coming to quick solutions. In retrospect, this was in some ways the easiest part of my life professionally. We were all working together: activists in the gay community, many of my gay friends who are now dead. But it was easy, in retrospect, because it was in the era of discovery. It is much harder now to face people who are not

xvi   *Preface: From the Grass Roots*

necessarily friends who are full of mistrust as we face the long haul. And the real challenge is all working together because none of us work together naturally, particularly on the long haul when there is so much uncertainty and it is so difficult.

These diverse and apparently contradictory perspectives warn us to listen closely and to think carefully before we create a history or judge a community. The epidemic is fractured. Our personal and organizational responses can cause further damage to the already injured. I believe that by understanding the sources and implications of these conflicting views, we can reduce that damage and strengthen our impact. If this work builds strength through knowledge and adds no harm, it will have accomplished all I hope from it.

Introduction

This book records a special aspect of the history of the AIDS epidemic: the way that poor people, people of color, gay men and lesbians, drug users, and women have built a social movement to oppose AIDS' devastating impact. Specifically, I have attempted to look at the ways that racism, sexism, and class have both limited and energized the responses of community organizations to the epidemic.

One of the most painful aspects of organizing is that, despite rhetoric and conscious attempts to respond to and keep biases and arrogance under control, these most human interferences to openness continually reassert themselves and prevent a clear view of the tasks and opportunities at hand. The organizations and movements documented in this book exhibit the working of both personal and institutionalized bias in community organizations. In some cases the struggle against this bias has been primarily internal to the organization; in others, a group has fought with policy makers or with other organizations.

Writing about the operation of bias within and among community organizations may sound like an attempt to discredit them. It is not. I hope that an explanation of the cultural and organizational sources of the often-present obstacles of racism and sexism will encourage a self-criticism that leads to change, not rigidity; a self-awareness that promotes a sympathetic understanding of oneself as well as others; and an ethical self-consciousness that assists in the transfer of skills and opportunities from the knowledgeable to those who do not know, and from the privileged to those who have been denied access to power.

AIDS dominated the political and social agenda of the gay movement throughout the eighties and continues to maintain its position as a primary focus in the nineties, especially for men. It is also a challenging class issue in feminist politics, a part of the struggle for African-American survival, a component of the emergence of Asian-American visibility, and a powerful force affecting de-criminalization attempts by prostitutes and drug users. Each "community," each individual approaches HIV in terms of an existing set of cultural norms and past experiences. The power relations within each group, among the groups, and between the groups and the dominant institutions are replayed (repeatedly) in the struggle against the epidemic.

The lessons to be learned from those damned by society to face the brunt of the epidemic include not only prescriptions for strategic inventions, but also conceptual and theoretical innovations. The strongest but least recognized innovations are those that have arisen from *praxis,* the dialectic between struggle and theorizing about that struggle. They are powerful because they are forged in practice. Pragmatic testing "in the street" can lead to intuitive development of folk wisdom.

When the traditional models of public health, epidemiology, and medicine are applied to the AIDS epidemic, they usually ignore the social organization of groups and look primarily at "interventions"—distribution of brochures, media campaigns, empowerment training, discussion groups, proper condom use. In contrast, I argue that the structures and processes of the groups are themselves keys to the success of the interventions, because it is organizational culture that ultimately determines who is served and how that service is accomplished.

This study of the AIDS epidemic draws on the literature of social movements and theories of bureaucracy. It examines the roles of race, gender, sexuality, and class in the creation of political agendas for the eighties and nineties. But this is also is a collection of stories. These are stories of organizations and networks formed by valiant women and men who tried to slow or stop an unstoppable epidemic. Some began their groups in lowly settings where those affected most by the epidemic met: a gay bar, a prostitute's home, around a kitchen table. Other organizations were dreamed up by health professionals and researchers in conference rooms and offices, sometimes just before a funding cycle. And still others were invented by community political activists and disillusioned liberals.

They include social movement organizations such as the Women's AIDS Network, of San Francisco, California, and New York City's ACT-UP;[1] the marginally legal Prevention Point needle exchange; the fiercely independent and street-focused California Prevention Education Project (Cal-PEP),[2] developed by African-American ex-prostitutes; and the struggling education projects of the Asian and Pacific Islander communities of Northern California. At the other end of bureaucratic stability is the San Francisco AIDS Foundation, one of the earliest AIDS organizations, founded in 1982 by predominantly white gay men.

These organizations represent a range of responses to the epidemic and reflect the diverse communities in which they are based. The organizational decisions made by their leaders over the past ten years, were informed by cultural values, community priorities, and economic opportunities and limitations, have produced both their strengths and their weaknesses. But what their varied existence demonstrates is that there is no one right answer for how to respond to AIDS.

Some AIDS response groups choose a focus on service; others are politically engaged. Some of the organizations are small or diffuse; others want to grow, but do not know how; still others have become nationally influential multi-million dollar bureaucracies. Issues of structure and process, hierarchy and democracy, professionalism and volunteerism have challenged them all.

Every group's work has been intricately embroidered (and sometimes beautifully elaborated) by its members' cultures and ideas about how one works with others. Cultural backgrounds are one key to an organization's structure, values, and goals. An example of cultural similarity within a group is the appeal of openly outrageous sexual expressiveness and camp shared by many white gay men. Such a sensibility marked the early days of the San Francisco AIDS Foundation and later flowered among ACT-UP activists. But these same white men also brought their sense of entitlement, including a belief in their right to "run" things and to define both history and current reality.

Alternatively, in San Francisco and Oakland, at the offices of the California Prostitute Education Project, there was an easy transition from street walker to street worker for the ex-prostitutes of Cal-PEP. But their cultural norms—dictated by what was necessary to survive on the streets—were to look after "family" members. Family includes co-workers in the prostitution business. This part of the prostitute culture was at odds with the traditional white, middle-class style of bureaucracy and was frequently described as inappropriate by other non-profits and funding agencies. Cal-PEP was disparaged in the press as ethically and legally suspect. Additionally, the external context of institutional racism, pre-existing funding priorities, and entrenched local and state political battles placed further constraints on this organization.

Although the epidemic and the number of related organizations continued to grow throughout the eighties, funding for research, prevention, and care stagnated and began to shrink under the Reagan and Bush administrations. Consequently, competition for resources has been intense, even when there has been an appearance of cooperation.

These organizations all began as movements for social change, but the majority inexorably developed in a direction that has made them increasingly similar to the bureaucracies and government agencies from which they initially wished to distinguish themselves. This process did not occur in exactly the same way or at the same rate for each of the organizations, and some organizations consciously chose to avoid institutionalization. Therefore, when they were forced to compete for scarce resources, the competition was often expressed as conflict over appropriate strategies. Thus organizations born in the intensity of community-based social movements have expanded into bureaucracies, only to find themselves under siege as part of the establishment they initially detested for its lack of concern.

Methodology: A Personal Approach

Where did this research begin? Perhaps when I first heard of AIDS. It was at a prison health conference sponsored by the American Medical Association in 1981 in Chicago.

It was the last day and time for a break. But the chair of the conference asked us to stay a minute. There was a special request from a representative from the medical service of the U.S. Bureau of Prisons. They had been seeing something new and wanted people to look out for it and report it to them if we saw it. They were afraid that there might be an epidemic (which to the Prison Health Service meant fifteen to twenty cases of a new disease) and it was new, but no one knew how serious at the time. The PHS speaker stepped to the podium and turned on slides. (I remember that slides were impressive to me then; I hadn't yet attended many medical conferences; now I know it's "their way.") There were pictures of red and purple Kaposi's Sarcoma lesions on white and black legs and perhaps elsewhere on the body.

(Was it an elbow? Those CDC slides of feet and legs and elbows that we used so much in the early days of AIDS education will haunt me forever. Did these come from the CDC civilian surveillance, or did the CDC get their originals from photos of these prisoners? It comes back to me again how often prisoners are the first to die, the last to be noticed. It is their condition to suffer and die, their great and only role in life.)

The speaker said that these lesions/this illness were turning up in more than one location. The PHS felt there might be some association with prisoners who were gay and/or IV drug users, but they didn't know exactly what the connection was.

The gay connection struck me because I had just heard a report at the conference of a study that found that gay men were often the victims of violence in prison, especially rape, and that the perpetrators were usually men who identified themselves as straight. The Bureau of Prisons' reaction to that study had been to suggest segregation of the gay men and/or restricting homosexuality in some way. This approach contrasted with what I thought was appropriate: to control the violence of the rapists. So part of my reaction to the possible gay connection to the new illness was that they would probably use this against gay men in prison. (Which did happen later.) Also, I thought, "Why would gay sex be associated with a rare illness like this?" Was it rape-related?

I knew, and the rest of the room knew, that it wasn't specifically a "gay" disease. No one who knew anything about prison could think that, because the prison pattern was broader than "gay" from the very start. I don't think that the Bureau of Prisons ever called AIDS "GRID."[3]

I had come to the prison health conference to watch and learn and share my own research. I was at the end of six years of increasingly focused study on women's health and health care in jails and prisons. I had begun to publish the results in various academic journals, to advocate for prisoners, and to act as an expert witness. I was preparing a book that would bring together my partial studies and incorporate further interviews and field notes. I thought it would all be done in a year or two, with perhaps a footnote or comparative comment to this new disease.

Instead, job politics intruded. In June 1982, I was denied tenure (the academic euphemism for "fired") because my work was too concerned with social issues.

My sabbatical disappeared, the prison book was put on hold, and in July 1983, I went to San Francisco to look for another job. It was not until four years later, in 1987, that I was reinstated at my university. The prison book is still unwritten, perhaps to be tackled some time in the future. But the move to San Francisco made it possible for me to meet the people and get to know the organizations that are described in these pages.

Within a month of my arrival in San Francisco, I joined the Women's AIDS Network, a loose organization of feminists who were involved in the epidemic. My own participation was stimulated by my belief that women with AIDS were overwhelmingly the same women I had met in jail after jail. Between 1983 and 1990 I was, at one time or another, an active member, the coordinator, a board member, and (many times) a task force participant in WAN. I continued to stay in touch with prison health issues, only now my jail and prison focus shifted from general health issues to AIDS discrimination, prevention, and care for incarcerated women.

Through the San Francisco AIDS Foundation, where I began working in 1984, and WAN, I was at the birth of the Association for Women's AIDS Research and Education (AWARE) at San Francisco General Hospital. This research project began with money to study HIV transmission in women. From the start it was funded to study prostitutes' infection rates. AWARE recruited the prostitute rights organization, COYOTE (Call Off Your Old Tired Ethics), with which I was already familiar because of their extensive work with women caught in the criminal justice system. COYOTE was also linked to WAN through one of its members. When Cal-PEP was invented, partially as a bridge between COYOTE and AWARE, I joined its board and stayed on until 1990.

One connection led to another. Being a specialist on women's health issues brought me in contact with various community coalitions, ethnically focused health services, and drug rehabilitation programs. Furthermore, as a lesbian and a feminist I could not help seeing what was happening to me and my lesbian co-workers at the hands of our gay brothers, who seemed to be lauding us on Monday and ignoring us on Tuesday.

Being a believer and participant in direct action projects since 1960, I was fascinated by the many strategies that AIDS activists and advocates have utilized to try, try, and try to get some effective attention directed at the epidemic. I had been a member (volunteer and paid) of the Student Non-Violent Coordinating Committee from 1961 to 1966, and I had continued to be active in anti-racism and affirmative action struggles in the seventies and eighties. In these and other movements I was and continue to be an enthusiastic participant in affinity groups, marches, and civil disobedience. So, naturally, I was curious about the work of ACT-UP and other AIDS advocacy groups. I hope that my past experiences with the cultural and structural obstinacy of racism have also sharpened the perspective of this book.

As a teacher, my primary job at the University of California, since 1973, has been to train students to be social activist intellectuals. Consequently, from 1984 to 1987, I brought organizing theories to my full-time AIDS work. Now that I am back in the university, I have wanted to theorize more about what I learned in the AIDS world. AIDS activities, nationally and internationally, are not just an "industry," as some detractors have argued.[4] Instead, I believe they constitute a new social world, with meanings, values, cultures, social and economic relations, families, entertainments, and philosophies. This study is partially an attempt to let the reader see this new world.

Because I have my own perspective, the sources of which are introduced above, I know that despite my attempts to be rigorously objective, I have inevitably introduced my own biases. The selection of organizations, the focus on particular turning points in their history, the requests to specific women and men to tell their stories—all these decisions and many more reflect my own interests and desires. I make no apology for this, and as part of my presentation I will be telling the reader my reasons for the selections. To temper my biases, I have tried to express them as clearly as I can, consider contradicting evidence, and let people other than myself tell as much of the story as possible. Consequently, wherever possible, I have utilized interview material, public speeches, and writing by important actors in the organizations and movements that are the focus of this work. I want the reader to hear the voices of people situated differently in regard to the epidemic, especially when their differences arise from class, ethnicity, race, culture, and sexuality. There is no one truth in the selections of data (observations, quotations, documentary sources), even though the selections are the logical strings that guide one's arguments and interpretation. Although I have not profiled Latino or Native American organizations in this study, I believe my methodology, which examines the role of culture, as well as the structural constraints of racism, sexism and class, can provide a model which can be applied in settings other than the ones I chose: African American, white, and Asian American groups. My choices were affected by time, familiarity, cost, convenience, and my desire to examine a manageable number of organizations with divergent interests and styles of work.

The data are drawn primarily from notes and documents I collected over a ten-year period (1982-1992). In some cases, the notes are the official minutes of a meeting; in other cases they are more sociological, recorded after a day of observation, work, meetings, or demonstrations. In addition, I interviewed and taped speeches of people who espouse the philosophies of the organizations studied. Several research assistants (including David Whittier in New York, Christine Wong and Wendy Chapkis in San Francisco) also did field work and interviews. Current and former members of Prevention Point and the director of a 1993-95 study of that organization (Sheigla Murphy) shared their own notes and research. I have also analyzed the content of health education material to uncover the values presented by the organizations which created them.

An unfolding chronology of the organizations will indicate their historical and political relationships. A comparative analysis of their growth, structure, and activities will demonstrate the patterns which link them as social formations both to each other and to broader social movements.

I know that some of what I say about these AIDS organizations may feel harsh. If we are to learn from our past, it is crucial that we examine it honestly in order to understand the potential replicability of both our successes and our errors. At some points I present the words of others and then provide a context to their speech. At other times my own voice is more explicit. I have tried throughout to render the voices and behaviors of others as I heard or saw them. Yet, the view of the epidemic presented in this book will always be mine. As so many writers begin, my thanks to those who've brought their truths to this work. The errors of selection, emphasis, and interpretation are mine.

Women's Histories
of AIDS

American constructions of race and sexuality are conveyed repeatedly in the world of AIDS prevention and politics, teaching the rules of normalcy and marginality in America. These rules are part of the ideological backbone of racism and gender oppression. They reinforce the psychological and social process of "othering" that continues to prevent democratic, tolerant, and peaceful life for all Americans. The impact is much greater than just the immediate effects.

Does discrimination exist within AIDS organizations? Obviously, yes. There are at least two types of discrimination involved. In some organizations, one sees the replication of the normative view of America; for example, repeated images of segregation in AIDS graphics directed at the heterosexual population. On the other hand, and complementing the first problem, there is the unequal and discriminatory distribution of resources on a racial, sexual, or class basis. The cultural backgrounds and work experience of policy makers and the leaders of AIDS organizations determine their selection of prevention, service, and political interventions as well as the ways in which they respond to sexism, racism, and class.

Nothing better epitomizes the multiple voices and visions of AIDS than women's experiences of the epidemic. Here race, class, sexuality, and gender all intersect and sometimes clash. The voices you will hear in this chapter are those of women, including myself, with varying perspectives on the epidemic.

These histories stand on equal footing, as each—to the extent that it is an honest rendering of the teller's memory—is the story as the woman telling it experienced it. Thus, each is a true, but very different history of women's organizing in response to the epidemic.

In some cases, the woman telling the story seems to say that her story is not just hers but *the* story. It is here that we can see the struggle to define reality as part of an activist impulse, and we see the story as an interactive mode between the teller and the audience. Ken Plummer, in *Telling Sexual Stories,* argues that stories are part of the political process, that they live in the flow of power.[1] To even be able to tell a story is to be able to claim a space for it and for the narrative and thus to empower oneself. When a new narrative is constructed, told, heard by an audience and understood, a new community, identity, and discourse are being created.

The stories and histories of women and AIDS are two sides of one process, a personal account and a public accounting. The audience is brought into the speaker's (or writer's) world not simply to present information within a commonly understood reality, but also to acquaint the listener with a new experience or way of thinking—about sex, gender, women, and HIV infection. Thus, the telling of the stories is a way in which women build community, change understandings, and argue for action. These women's histories of the AIDS epidemic document the diversity of women with HIV/AIDS, while presenting opinions about the resistance of physicians and medical researchers to shifts in a male-centered paradigm that would incorporate their women-specific needs.

The "First National Scientific Meeting on HIV Infection in Adult and Adolescent Women" was held in Washington, D.C., in February of 1995. That the "first" national conference on women and AIDS was held so recently speaks eloquently to women's official exclusion, even as the number of cases among women was rapidly increasing.[2] From the very first address and throughout the conference, the dominant theme was that women had been given seriously short shrift in AIDS research and treatment, and even in the very definition of the disease. Here is Rae Lewis-Thornton, an African American woman with HIV who had recently been profiled in *Essence* magazine.

> [They say]: "Women don't become HIV-infected." The medical community has arrogantly been unkind to women, not just about AIDS, but with most diseases. They've excluded us from studies. And I speak from personal experience. I have been in a study at the National Institute of Health for nine years, and in the nine years of this study they have never taken a pelvic exam. If the medical community had indeed been sensitive and recognized that women, too, become HIV-infected, then in the earlier days could you imagine how much data we could have collected on HIV infection in women, if women had been included in the early designs of HIV studies? It's a sad thought. Government institutions, they've not only been in denial, but they have denied us. We have had to validate each other, prop each other up, and continue the fight. We have had to do that even when it was unpopular and even when we were the only voices in the wilderness.[3]

The women HIV affects are more varied than the virus's own mutations. The following voices of women demonstrate the radically different AIDS histories of those who are situated in different social locations: the centers of federal power, the heartlands of radical activism, marginalized ethnic or sexual communities, or within academic and research institutions. These various histories of the epidemic constitute a multi-focal view that is a key to women's multiple interventions (in both a theoretical and a practical sense) in the epidemic.

No matter how great the differences between the women who speak, they are united by the fact that they have had to struggle in order to gain recognition for women with AIDS. Mary Lucey, an ACT-UP member, discovered the epidemic and her own infection simultaneously.

> For a lot of years, like a lot of women, I lived an unconscious life when it came to issues concerning HIV and AIDS. It's not something I'm proud of, but it's true. Like so many of us I was content to seek the shelter of my own little world. I didn't just wake up one day and decide to become an AIDS activist. I came from the depths of a living hell, the same hell that many of you have lived through. I paroled in 1989, got strung out, got pregnant, and got HIV.
>
> I tested positive while I was pregnant. When I tried to find services and medical care the response was the same everywhere I went. It seemed that no one in Los Angeles had ever seen a woman with HIV before. I was referred in a circle of agencies, always ending up at the same one, the one with women and AIDS in their title. But they had never encountered any women who actually had HIV infection, and they didn't know what to do with me either. Everyone wanted to write a story about me. They wanted to take my picture, they wanted to interview me for the 11 o'clock news. But no one wanted to provide me with medical care. No one seemed to know where I could find a doctor . . . .
>
> AIDS is a political disease. There is much more to this disease than simply what we experience as individuals on a day-by-day basis. Living daily with this virus in our bodies is a tremendous thing to deal with, yet there is more. There is the part you may not see every day. It's almost hidden at times, but it's there—the politics that control our lives and influence our very survival. The only way we can begin to make anything better for any one of us is to try to make things better for all of us. We dare not let an entire generation of women die. We dare not let AIDS become an accepted part of women's lives. We must rethink our strategy for survival. We must never accept that our government did nothing to stop AIDS from spreading. We are not talking about sex and morality. We are talking about a deadly virus. We're talking about fighting for our lives.

Mary Lucey's history of AIDS is chilling. As late into the epidemic as 1989, women were still invisible to providers of medical and social services to people with AIDS. By 1995, there had been some change, but the struggle was still going on to have women included in the very definition of AIDS by the Centers for Disease Control (CDC).

Even Patricia Fleming, director of the Office of National AIDS Policy and the government's spokesperson at the 1995 conference, concedes that women's history in the epidemic was one of unrelenting marginalization. Fleming, African-American, heterosexual, well-educated, and well-connected, speaks from the center of policy formation. Her phrasing emphasizes that she is also a woman, like those with HIV. But the phrasing is disinguous when it obscures the fact that HIV among women is a disease of the poor, the uneducated, and the ghetto-ized. Her assertion of gender commonality confuses the situation instead of clarifying it.

Let's be frank. For much of this epidemic many of our needs were ignored or shoved aside by government leaders who cared either too little or cared not at all. Women were and still are misdiagnosed or not diagnosed at all, and women were woefully under-represented in clinical trials of AIDS therapies. The CDC AIDS case definition didn't recognize our symptoms or our illnesses, and Social Security didn't pay for our dis-abilities, and no natural history study was tracking the course of our infections . . . .

I remember working with Maxine Wolfe years ago, fighting for changes in [the Department of] Health and Human Services. I'm pleased to say that we've made some remarkable progress. Working together we've opened the doors that were shut in our faces; and the remarkable thing is that many of those who were on the other side of those doors are now glad we pushed so hard, because we helped them to do things they wanted to do but found it difficult to accomplish. The changes we have won have broad implications for women with other conditions and diseases . . . .

We can grumble about how long it's taken, but let's also look at how far we've come. Just in the past few years women's health in general and women in HIV in particular are taken more seriously and are a top priority in the federal government. We've seen some very important changes in the areas of AIDS research and drug development. NIH (National Institutes of Health) now has an affirmative policy requiring the inclu-sion of women and racial and ethnic minorities in all clinical trials, including those for AIDS. That's an important change and one we should all be proud of. NIH has created the Office of Research and Women's Health, and women's committees now exist with-in the AIDS clinical trials group and the community programs for clinical research on AIDS. The FDA, in response to the advice of the National Task Force on AIDS Drug Development, has improved its own guidelines on the inclusion of women in clinical trials by pharmaceutical companies.

Almost a decade—too long—after the men's natural history study was begun, NIH launched a women's inter-agency HIV study to identify the nature and rate of HIV dis-ease progression in women. NIH has established a program of research specific to women with AIDS, including opportunistic infections, malignancies, and neurological manifestations. This year NIH will devote more than $260,000,000 to this AIDS research specific to women.

Fleming went on to detail other gains for women infected with HIV within the CDC, NIH, the Office of AIDS Research, and other agencies of government. But the speaker who followed her, Maxine Wolfe, a long-time member of New York City ACT-UP, took a decidedly different approach to the same history. Wolfe is a white lesbian and an academic, with an extensive history of radical activism prior to and during the epidemic.

I agreed to speak today because I feel a special responsibility to people I have worked with most closely who aren't alive to tell their versions of this history. It's to them—par-ticularly to Katrina Haslip, Iris de la Cruz, Lydia Awadalla, Tamar Sokel, as well as to Ortiz Alderson, Robert Garcia, Charlie Barber, and Lee Shy—that it is dedicated, and it's also dedicated to Keri Duran, whose picture is down there, who planned to be here today but was too sick to travel. It's a history in which lesbians, heterosexual women, and gay men, infected and uninfected, from diverse cultural and economic circum-stances and life experiences, have worked together. So it contradicts the myths that say we can't and the rumors that say we haven't. It's a history with names, though there is no way I can include everyone in it. It's not about abstract numbers or statistics, but about real people, some of whom fought for women's lives and some of whom didn't. It's a history that won't be found in government press releases.

My history of women and AIDS is a history of criminal neglect by a government and its agencies, including those charged with public health and treatment research. It's a history of unscientific and unethical research, of white male science, of indifference to women. It's also a history of racism, sexism, classism, homophobia, addictophobia, and paternalism. It's a history in which researchers, medical practitioners, and government representatives feel perfectly okay calling the women in their research studies "the moms" and have acted publicly as if the fact that a woman is HIV infected, poor, a woman of color, a drug user, an ex-inmate, or a lesbian means that we are too stupid to understand the world or the choices we have to make. Instead they, the experts and the politicians, want us to let them make the decisions for us.

In 1982 an article published in the *Annals of Internal Medicine* reported on opportunistic infections in five previously healthy women, all of whom had been diagnosed in 1981. One was described as a bisexual who did not use injection drugs, one was described as a heterosexual who did not use injection drugs but who had a male sexual partner who did, three were described as injection-drug users who were heterosexual. Three women were Latinas, one was African American, and one was white. One woman had symptoms for thirty-four months before she got one of the opportunistic infections the Centers for Disease Control had identified with the illness that would eventually be called AIDS, infections they had found in gay white men. It was reported that one woman had swollen lymph nodes in her cervix, and one had bacterial pneumonia, symptoms it would take another ten years for the government to admit might be connected to AIDS.

For years the Centers for Disease Control, the National Institutes of Health, and every other government agency, as well as the medical research and treatment establishments and the media, chose to make us invisible. And even though we are far more likely to be infected by others than to infect others, when they made us visible, we were and still are treated as vectors of transmission to men and to fetuses . . . .

It was ten years into this epidemic and eight years after that first article before the U.S. government sponsored a conference on Women and HIV/AIDS, and even getting a conference was a battle . . . .[4]

At that conference, which took place in December 1990, Dr. Fauci, the head of the National Institute of Allergy and Infectious Diseases, was given the opportunity to address the almost 1,500 attendees at a plenary session like this. Since neither he nor his agency had done any research about women and AIDS, he was using his time to give us an AIDS 101 lecture, telling us how the virus worked. Tamar Sokel from Women Fighting AIDS felt compelled to interrupt him. She stepped up to the microphone and told him in no uncertain terms that the only degree she had was one in "streetology" but she, and every other infected woman she knew, knew how the virus worked. When some of the attendees, most of whom worked in AIDS service organizations, started yelling at her to let him speak, she told them that if they didn't know how the virus worked, they should resign from their jobs; it was a waste of her time . . . .

Twenty-five women identified themselves as women with HIV and read a statement they had written. They demanded that the Centers for Disease Control change the definition of AIDS to include infections women with HIV get, that the disability regulations be changed so that women could get disability based on the infections they got, and that women have access to research studies to potentially life-saving treatment.

At that same conference, women demonstrated against Dr. James Curran of the Centers for Disease Control, who was still insisting that the definition of AIDS could be changed to include infections women get, but there wasn't enough evidence. One woman after another interrupted him to give him evidence. They told him about their infections, cervical cancer, bacterial pneumonia, pelvic inflammatory disease, yeast infections. He claimed the CDC was funding research that they weren't funding, so some researchers and doctors had to get up and contradict him.

Only one month earlier, women AIDS activists had met with Dr. Gary Noble, who was then head of HIV at the Centers for Disease Control, and with epidemiologists on their staff. We had presented them with lots of data. It was clear to us that their position did not stem from ignorance. All they could say was that changing the definition would upset their statistics, make Congress suspect their motives, and make white middle-class women with yeast infections nervous.

The double standard was apparent. For example, the previous definition of AIDS in gay men had not been based on rigorous, controlled scientific research. That definition had been based on reports from clinicians. Yet the CDC said that thirty-three studies showing a relationship between immune suppression and cervical cancer weren't enough because there was no definite causal link. Katrina Haslip was at that meeting. Katrina was a central figure in the AIDS Counseling and Education, or ACE, project when she was in Bedford Hills Prison . . . . She said in response to their statements, "I hold you personally responsible for the deaths of every woman from HIV, including myself."

And Katrina did die without an AIDS diagnosis, although she had had multiple bouts of bacterial pneumonia and lots of other types of infections. But she lived long enough to see the CDC definition changed.

Getting to that point took two years of intense activism. The CDC Campaign included every strategy and tactic there is, beginning with a demonstration in Atlanta at the CDC headquarters in January 1990. A second large demonstration was held in December 1990, only a couple of weeks before the Women in HIV Conference. At that demonstration many women with HIV marched for miles and held a public speakout despite the most torrential downpour I have ever seen. Katrina was there, Lydia, Tamar, Iris de la Cruz; it was there that I met Mary Lucey and Keri Duran. I remember sitting on the steps outside of the jail having a conversation with Mary Lucey about her continuing vaginal discharge, one of the only ways women had to get and share information as late as 1990 . . . .

Local actions about changing the definition took place all over the country. There was an ACT-UP petition and postcard campaign, and petition campaigns were started by all different groups, from the grassroots all over the country. Despite all of this, the Centers for Disease Control twice tried to release a new definition which would not include women's or drug users' infections. Each time, we wrote critiques, mailed them out all over the country, urging people to send in public comment . . . . The CDC received 12,000 letters of public comment about their idea of a definition, and it didn't matter.

When they made their second attempt to change the definition, we asked people to send letters to their Senators and Representatives demanding a public investigation of the CDC. So they backed down again . . . .

The CDC campaign also included pressuring for and testifying at national and local hearings in which activists would constantly have to counter knowingly-presented misinformation from the Centers for Disease Control. Confrontations with James Curran and Gary Noble took place at the International Conference in Amsterdam, where AIDS activists from the United States were joined by women from all over the world, because the World Health Organization used the CDC AIDS definition.

The campaign also included sending out media packets. Robin Hatter and Laurie Cotter did so much of that work, and it resulted in hundreds of newspaper articles, spearheaded by the ones written by Elinor Burkett of the *Miami Herald*, articles in which for the first time in the public media women's symptoms were described.[5] There was also a full page ad in the *New York Times* with a headline that said, "Women don't get AIDS, they just die from it," and 300 groups from across the country signed onto it. Coming behind all of that work, four years of work, we pulled together a coalition of women from different groups and we finally forced the CDC to hold a public hearing in the fall of 1992.

Then we also had to force them to invite the doctors and the researchers who were seeing women and had the information. They only wanted the CDC researchers to speak, who we knew would give the government line again. Then we had to raise $20,000 so that infected women who couldn't afford it could attend, something the government was unwilling to do. Then we had to get the media there, which we did.

At the end of that hearing and after four years of work, and even though he had no more information than he had in the beginning, Dr. Curran finally had to admit that he had been convinced to add three clinical conditions to the CDC definition of AIDS: bacterial pneumonia, TB, and stage-three cervical cancer, and to add recurrent vaginal candidiasis to the category of HIV symptomatic.

When Katrina found out that the CDC was going to change the definition, she was in the hospital near death. In fact, she died only a short time later. Yet, when a reporter asked her how she felt about the fact that the government had changed the definition of AIDS, she answered, "The government didn't change the definition of AIDS—we did—we did! And it's not enough! We want and need more." And we do.

If women in general have been made invisible in the AIDS epidemic, lesbian women have fared even worse. Here is the story that Tara, a California lesbian of Native American heritage, told me in 1989.[6] I quote this interview almost in its entirety because it is so vivid as a history of a lesbian and a woman of color with AIDS.

So I was really sick and emotionally really flipping out, and I was having trouble working. So I stopped working and all of a sudden had no income, and everything was starting to fall apart, and all of a sudden my relationship broke up, too. So I was more or less headed towards a nervous breakdown. And I was getting sicker, like really bad lung infections, and I'd lost about thirty pounds in two months. My glands were swollen, and I went, "Wow, God. I'm really sick. I wonder what this is?" And so I went to a doctor on my way out of town, because I was going to go to LA to try to save my sanity. And the doctor sort of asked me all these questions about AIDS, possible risks, and I was like, "It's stress. I'm just under a lot of stress. It's stress." So my denial was severe.

I got to LA, and by the time I got to LA they were like putting oxygen on me on the airplane. They'd given me a TB test and my arm was like out to here. I was just coughing up blood, and weighed 109 pounds, and called a cab and went to the friend's house where I was going to stay and they looked at me and they said, "My god, what the hell is wrong with you? What are you doing here?" You know? And so they took me to a hospital. I spent twenty-four hours in a hallway on a gurney with a 106° fever. They wouldn't let me take the antibiotics that I had, to try to control the lung infection that I had. They had all of their shit hung up all over these curtains around me saying gloves and everything because they thought I had TB, although my x-ray showed that I didn't, that what I had was pneumonia. But basically they were real reactionary. I saw a doctor for about two minutes. I saw fifteen medical students. All of them spent at least fifteen minutes poking and prodding me. They collapsed every vein that they could get to in this arm, half of the ones in this arm, when I finally just said, "I'm not having anybody else touch me."

So [after] about fifteen hours of this [within a] twenty-four hour period, by this time I'm scared shitless and these guys are coming in here—and they were all men—and they were just completely oblivious. It's like as if I was not there. And they're talking to each other about, "Wow. We're finally going to get to work with an AIDS patient." And I'm lying there going, "No, I don't have—no, no, no. I'm stressed out. No." But [I'm] in a hallway, eight-hundred miles away from home, with a broken heart and knowing that I'm getting ready to move, and I have no money because I can't work.

How I agreed to take the AIDS test was that I hadn't eaten in about fifteen hours and they hadn't changed my sheets or my gown since I got there, and it was drenched. I mean I had a 106° fever still, and they hadn't done anything to bring my fever down either. So I agreed that I would sign their little paper to let them give me this test if they would just feed me and change my bed linens. So they wanted to take this test. They were just like hoping for that, so they brought me some food and changed my gown and then left me there when I threw it back up, and I had to sit there for fifteen minutes. I finally just threw it in a pile and threw it in the hallway and let it splash against the wall, which flipped them out, because they had me in isolation curtains. And I just figured, hey, if you're going to treat me like shit I'm going to give it back to you.

They wouldn't let me make any phone calls, they wouldn't let me get a hold of anybody. And finally I snuck out and I called my friends and they came and kidnapped me from the hospital. And I immediately started feeling better. They also stole my meds back for me, my antibiotics.

But they already had my phone number of where I was staying, and two days later—I mean I'm still, literally, having a nervous breakdown and flipping out and heartbroken and trying to figure out what I'm going to do—I get this phone call from this doctor who's supposedly treated me. I only have vague memory of him. Calls me up and he says, "Well, your test came back. You're positive. You have AIDS. If not AIDS, you at least have severe ARC and we want you to check right back in." And I, more or less I lost it, and I told him where he could stick his diagnosis. I told him that I felt like it was the most severe medical abuse that I could even conceive.

And that's kind of where it started. So eight-hundred miles away from home, absolutely no counseling, no type of sensitivity whatsoever . . . . I started trying to get a hold of AIDS organizations to support me, who were all basically run by gay men, and they worked really well as far as gay men went, and their response to me was like, "What the hell do you want? I don't know that there's anything that we can do for you. We don't have any lesbian-specific services. We don't really even have any women-specific services, so call this place and call this place."

Once I knew that I had a diagnosis, I knew that I had a choice. I could either choose to live or I could choose to die, and I knew that anything in between was choosing to die. So I went to a hypnotherapist and it was like, God, I've got a lot of shit in here, a lot of the shit that says I don't deserve to live. So what are we going to do about this? So I sort of took a crash course in changing my attitudes about myself and about how I felt about my life and came back ready to take it by the horns. And I knew that I had to come back up here and deal with the shit. It was like this is where the shit started; this is where it was going to get worked through. So I had to come back here.

When I got back up here, the first thing I wanted to do was just like join a support group. Meet another woman. Find another lesbian—I didn't even think another one would exist, even though I was really active. I mean I'd been working for three years really closely and had experienced at least 30 deaths, like holding the hands of someone while they die. So I was so close to it, but I had not met another woman yet. Which surprised me, considering that I've been doing feminist action for a really long time. But I'm sure that my denial had a lot to do with it.

Tara, like many other lesbians, had been active as a volunteer in the battle against the epidemic. Therefore, she was familiar with the resources the Bay Area had to offer and attempted to access them.

When I came up here to get services, financially I was in really bad shape, so I went to any place that I thought might give me financial help. And I was familiar with all of these services. I can't tell you how many people I drove to these services, held their hands and bitched for them so they could get it, because they weren't strong enough to do it for themselves. And here I was, really sick, having a nervous breakdown. Only it was getting worse, and I was starting to have some real severe memory loss.

I was doing things like writing down my phone number and address so that I could find my way home. Writing a list of like "Brush your teeth and comb your hair before you leave the house," because I'd leave the house and realize it's like, God, I'm wearing the shirt I woke up in which was still sticky from sweating in. I mean I was really not okay. But I was still attempting to go to these services, and I couldn't find any support. I couldn't find anybody to go to these services with me. And the response that I got was mostly, the gay male response is, "You're supposed to be taking care of us." And I knew a lot of these people. I had been taking care of them for three years, and they were turning around as if I was betraying them, somehow, by being sick. And I'm standing there going, "God damn it, I've done it for three years. I want it back now." And their resistance was like, I think their denial was about, "No, no, no. Don't you guys cave in on us. You're valuable. Don't get sick, too." But I was too emotionally distraught and too physically ill to be able to advocate for myself at that point or to get outraged directly. All I could do was walk away more overwhelmed. And I sort of picked up the philosophy: If I could just hold on long enough, just hold on long enough . . .

And so I went like that for weeks, getting crazier, losing my personality basically, and getting sicker. I'd lost all the weight that I'd gained while I was in LA, and I was getting another lung infection. And my lymphadenopathy was getting really bad. And finally I just completely lost it.

A friend of mine found me underneath my dining room table huddled up in a ball, soaking wet and hysterical. And she took me to this place called Mission Crisis, which was just like County Mental Health, and dumped me in the lap of a woman that works with people with HIV disease. Who also happened to be a lesbian. How my friend managed to do this so well, I'm not sure, because she had no idea. She was just like, "I've got to take her somewhere because she's not going to survive." So this woman pulled some strings for me. It's like that's what it took for me as a woman to get some help, which I find just completely inadequate and unacceptable. I know that maybe most cases are not that extreme. But, if one person goes through that, it's too extreme. And most of the women that I know have had real similar experiences in terms of getting to complete desperation before they can get any help.

In any case, it got me connected with the San Francisco AIDS Foundation, and I joined a group for women that were HIV-positive in which I was the only lesbian, and I also was the only person that was not immediately struggling with IV drug use. So I went out in search of other services, services that were for women who weren't IV drug users, or educational services, or medical services. Any service that I could possibly get my hands on.

What I found was that basically there are no women's services. There's little parts of "Well, we also have this person that does women's programs," but as far as organizationally, the services are very limited. And then, just about all the funds that they get are directed to IV drug users, because it's the biggest population with women.

As a lesbian that meant that there were absolutely no services. Nothing that was geared toward my needs, which are different from straight women. Not crucially, it's not that I can't use women's services; I'm a woman, I can. However, support systems. I couldn't understand why there weren't any for lesbians. I kept being told that there were like twelve lesbians in San Francisco that were HIV-positive. I later found out that it was more like ten. And I wanted to know how come all ten of them weren't getting together as a support group? How come we didn't know each other? How come none of them knew each other? And how come three quarters of them wouldn't tell their true names when they got services? Well, then I found out. Then I found out.

I decided that, damn it, if there's no services for us, then I'm going to create them. That I'm going to find a way to get these women to come together, and then I'm going to find a way to get the lesbian community to acknowledge that we're here and to help us.

The response pretty much in the lesbian community is very similar to my denial, that we don't get it. And then we're so burned out from working on it, it's like don't bring it home, too. We have to deal with this everywhere; the only place we don't have to deal with this is right here, in our own personal space. And I'm standing up and going, "No, gotta deal with it there, too." And so I just got hit with incredible resistance.

And I'd say that the main breakthrough in terms of me deciding to organize and deciding how I was going to go about that was that I heard about a "Lesbian Caregivers and the AIDS Epidemic" conference. And I went there, I was invited to do a workshop, a panel workshop, with a few other women, on lesbians at risk professionally and personally. And these are caregivers, so these are like lots of nurses that get stuck all the time and that do deal with professional risk.

And we went through most of this workshop, and there's like twenty minutes left in this workshop, and I had already sort of been stepping on toes about, "It's here. It's here." Because they were like just, "No, no, no. No, no, no."

And I finally said, "Wow. We've been talking about it all this time, and any time we get near anything that's personal, everybody changes it back to professional. I feel like we've covered that really well, and I want to talk about your personal risks." And so I talked a little about myself and started making jokes, making cracks. Through the whole thing, pretty much, I was making cracks about some of the things that they were talking about.

Well, when we started talking about personal risk, and I started challenging their ideas. I realized, "Wow. This is severe."

Some of them were resisting, they got mad at me. They said, "You're an isolated case. What are you talking about?" I'm going, "I'm not an isolated case. I'm here. And it's happening, and it's growing, and more of us are getting infected."

I was the only person in the entire room besides one other person that was interested in safe sex among lesbians. It just was like, "Women don't give it to each other." Bullshit. We bleed. We have risk. And especially the lesbian community.

So anyway, when the conference got back together there was this whole room and it was "Strategizing for the Future." Like what's the next step, as lesbians? What are we going to do next? And these women are talking about all this stuff that's removed from them. I mean we're talking about lesbian health care and trying to create an agenda so that we get our needs met, because basically the reality is that the lesbian community has been involved in creating the model for the AIDS health care system.

In a big way, what happened was gay men saw our model and saw that the feminist model of health care worked. And they jumped on our bandwagon. And as time progressed and the epidemic grew, we got bumped off. And so women's health care has just plummeted. And so now women's health care basically is a real individualized thing . . . .

And so these women are getting mad. We're starting to go, "Okay. It's time to take care of ourselves again. Not at the exclusion of men, but it's time for us to jump back on the bandwagon. We put a lot of effort in; now we want some of the rewards, too."

Well, that seemed a really good place to talk about lesbians and AIDS, and when I started talking—and mind you, I was the only woman at this entire conference of like two-hundred women that identified herself as HIV-positive. I don't know if there were others. I just know that nobody else spoke up, and so that was severely isolating in itself.

But this response was like, "Now wait a minute. So lesbians and AIDS. But we have this whole other agenda going on. One in three women gets cancer." And I'm going, "Yeah, and we've got to work on that. That's really scary, too. But it's like this hasn't even been addressed." And women got really angry at me. The denial was so severe. And at one point I was even told, "You've had your chance to talk. Lots of other people would like to talk." What I wanted to do was get it out there, and I wanted to step on some toes.

I wanted to make people realize that none of us are just safe by virtue of our sexual identification or anything else. And one of the things that I did was, I stood up there and I said, "How many of you have never had sex with a man? And how many of you have never done drug use?" It's like most of the women in this room are somewhere between twenty-five and forty. It's like the era you grew up in. "How many of you never once did an IV drug? How many of you never had anal sex with a guy when you were still seeing guys?" Most of us started somewhere. And then, "How many of you really believe that lesbians never have sex with men?" And I finished it with, "How many of you really believe that lesbians don't lie?"

And I'm not condemning the lesbian community, because I'm really proud of the action that the lesbian community has taken on, but it doesn't mean that we are enlightened about health care or about our own needs or our own risks. The women's community has rampant sexually transmitted diseases in our community right now. Why? Because everyone's screwing everybody, and no one's paying attention. And no one realizes how much on the rise a lot of these infections are. And no one's interested in safe sex because we're lesbians, we don't need it. And that's what I was there to confront.

I had lots of women walk up to me and say, just in the process of me coming out as a woman with AIDS, walk up to me and say, "Well, what did you do? Fuck a man?" And it's like, "Well, does that make me less of a lesbian if I did?" However, I had to defend against that, that I was not a good lesbian because I had this disease, and that I was betraying my community, and I was betraying women as a whole. I got the same shit from straight women. What did I *do?* I must have done *something* wrong. If a gay man gets this infection, and he stands up and says, "And 4,000 other of my brothers are in this with me." A woman stands up and says, "My God, I don't want to tell anybody because they're going to condemn me." The average woman tells two people. The average lesbian tells less . . . .

And so I decided that it needed to be taken off a personal level and onto a political level. And so what I did was, I'd remembered the names—actually I had written them all down—of women who were somewhat supportive of the things that I had said at this conference. And so I called these women. All of them either directors or very active in the services, like Judith Stevenson, Executive Director of Operation Concern, Jackie Hansen and Geni Bowie from the Mid-City Consortium on AIDS, and a couple other women. And I told them what had happened. And they got really mad, too. And I said, "So let's get together and do something."

And so we pulled these women together and decided that what we wanted to do was focus on safe sex education for lesbians, for women in general. We wanted to be confrontive in terms of agencies that weren't offering services for women and agencies that had absolutely no possible services for lesbians. It seems really inappropriate to have therapists for women and then have no lesbian therapists who are available to work with women, because they're so booked up working with men. It's like, well, free 'em up. Make the priority. It has to happen.

Basically what I feel is that lesbian health care has taken a back burner to AIDS care, and we're not included in that. Health care is inaccessible; the services are inaccessible. I tried to get into Quan Yin's AIDS Alternative Healing Program and it was over $4,000 for six months! I don't even make $4,000 a year now. So maybe gay men can pull that together.

But what I want is for gay men to fund me joining that program. I've been taking care of them. And even if I hadn't been taking care of them, my community has. And so those are my goals—to rally the gay male community. Not turn against them or turn them against us. We were there when they needed us. Now things are turning around. One in three women have breast cancer or some form of cancer. The death rate is incredible. And then AIDS cases, the number of deaths and the number of women who are HIV-positive is phenomenal considering what it was three years ago. So all I want, my intention, and the intention of this group that I've formed is to rally support . . . .

I feel like women in general are pretty much in denial around our needs, our own agendas. We deny that we don't have adequate health care, and then we deny that we really deserve to put that ahead of an agenda like AIDS, that we actually deserve to do it at the same time. Because basically if we don't survive, what the hell good does it do to support the men's community, either? And AIDS support basically is male—whether it's gay or not, the AIDS support systems are basically directed around men.

When Tara told her story, there were no organizations of women with HIV. Women Organized to Respond to Life-threatening Disease (WORLD) had not yet been formed. A year later, in 1990, this organization of HIV-positive women was developed in the San Francisco Bay area. It began to publish its monthly newsletter that highlights personal histories of women with HIV, updates on medical treatments, and events of interest. The organization's board is all HIV- positive. It sponsors retreats and other events for women and their families, and promotes local, regional, national, and international advocacy for women. It began when its founder Rebecca Denison could find no support groups which matched her needs. She brought her background as a political activist in Central America to the task of creating an organization for women. While WORLD is not specifically for lesbians, it includes lesbians in a non-judgmental way. It also represents the multifaceted organizing approach found in some men's organizations, but missing in most services directed at women by mainstream organizations. But even WORLD was not an organization for lesbians with HIV.

The women who have spoken so far in this chapter have told very different stories of the epidemic, but these differences are not contradictions. Each story is an attempt to find understanding and create a response. Each view is accurate as a reflection of the subjective experience of the reporter. Patricia Fleming and Maxine Wolfe both see themselves as feminists and active in the struggle against sexism in AIDS policies. But while one sees progress and cooperation, the other sees conflict and struggle. Each identifies herself as a true voice for women. While Tara and Rae Lewis-Thornton both see the history of AIDS in personal terms, Tara's account is painful; for her, a broad inclusive history is less important than immediate activism. Rae, as the opening speaker at a conference on women and HIV, is critical and optimistic. Histories are inaccurate only when they make assertions about others' experiences or assume that others who share our identity or location vis-à-vis the epidemic have experiences similar to our own.

The next voice you hear is my own, speaking as an AIDS activist, a sociologist, a lesbian, and a feminist. When I first wrote this section, I had already published several "histories" of the AIDS epidemic that focused on women. One chronicled the start of the epidemic in northern California and the need for services,[7] a second the growth of individualized empowerment programs and their inevitable limitations.[8] Another detailed the spread of the epidemic and the types of illnesses which women get;[9] and in still a different approach, I constructed an account that described the key issues for feminist strategizing on a global level.[10] These were all biography and history, each constructed for a special purpose and reflecting my education, my social location within the epidemic and in the broader society, and the audience for whom I had a particular message. In the specific history I have chosen to repeat in this book, the first decade of the epidemic is retold through the story of lesbian activists. Although their experiences are not so different from other women's involvement, there is a special connection that arises from their "homosexual" linkage to the epidemic. This story includes my own history but it is primarily a sociological analysis of feminist and lesbian AIDS activism in the 1980s. To more fully understand this activism, it is useful to first visit the seventies, during which gay and lesbian cultures emerged in new forms. This digression also provides a background for other struggles described later.

The combination of the second wave of feminism and the emergence of the gay liberation movement in the seventies led to a complex flowering of culture and social organization by women.[11] Many of the leadership roles in the women's movement were filled by lesbians (part-time, occasional, emerging, temporary, long-term, and otherwise). This was a mutual love affair by lesbians for feminism (the idea that women matter) and of feminism for the essence of the lesbian vision (women come first in time, emotional interest, and political commitment). The slogan that "feminism is the theory and lesbianism the practice" may not be perfectly true, but its emotional validity brought the two movements together. In addition, most feminist organizations during this period attempted to include both heterosexuals and lesbians. On the subject of the body, the motto of feminism was "our bodies, our selves," which was not just a health slogan but also a call for self-determination, expressed in forms ranging from self-examination to sexual experimentation. Lesbians became leaders in many of the feminist institutions formed in the seventies.

In many cases, the language of the movement itself conflated women and lesbians. During the mid-seventies, for example, as lesbian culture went public, it was labeled "women's culture" by its promoters, *viz.* "women's music," which was really, of course, lesbian music, and music for a predominantly white and college-educated audience at that.

The feminist movement and the lesbian movement were parallel and interconnecting. But they were also linked to other movements and had considerable diversity within them, which is often lost in the telling.[12] There is a widespread notion that the "women's movement" was white and middle-class,[13] but as I experienced it, it was intentionally cross-class and multiracial. Feminists and lesbians in all segments of the population were active in prison reform and organizing, battered women's shelters, anti-racist organizing, ethnic liberation struggles, school board fights, and reproductive rights that addressed sterilization abuse.[14]

Despite some invisibility in the eyes of the white left and to many white gay men, it was during the seventies that both lesbians and women (at least the feminists in the name of women) "went public."[15] Gaining experience in their own movements as well as other struggles, they began to create new sets of institutions for women. As a result, for lesbians, new organizations emerged beyond women's bars and the sports clubs associated with them. Suddenly separatist settings and services for women (health clinics, therapy services, restaurants, bookstores,

retreats, land groups, classes, caucuses) were everywhere. Women's studies cours-
es and programs were invented. Gay and straight women mingled. Lesbianism
was presented as a legitimate option for women; many lesbian-inclined women
chose it and did so openly in ways that their older sisters could not have done so
easily.

Feminism helped make this development of women's "spaces" and lesbian
lifestyle and culture possible, because it brought the energies of women of all sexual persuasions together in the name of "women," therefore making available
many more resources than either straight women or lesbians could generate by
themselves. Each group had access to different types of resources. In a certain way,
the reason why lesbians have led the women's movement and its institutions is
that lesbians have more labor, more focused attention, and less distraction to
offer: they are not so torn by the need to return home to men. On the other hand,
the connections of straight women to men brought a different set of resources,
especially financial aid. Because women's salaries ranged from 59 percent to 63
percent of men's during this period, a woman with a man was likely to live in a
wealthier household than a woman with a woman.

The movement for gay liberation, which emerged as a powerful force in 1969
and spread internationally within a few years, further affected lesbian visibility,
politics, economics, and culture. While men dominated the movement, women
were assertive in many of its political organizations and other institutions. The
movement's effects on lesbian-gay solidarity varied by location: in larger urban
areas, men dominated the economy and the institutions of the gay community;
socializing by men and women was predominantly segregated and reflected different sexual, political, and social values.

Lesbian culture, in both its older and its new institutions, was characterized by
a more socially critical stance—beyond lesbian/gay assertion. Because women
had fewer institutions to call their own, their gathering places continued to be
more mixed in terms of race and class than did male institutions. Gay men's institutions, on the other hand, were more likely to replicate the class and race character of the larger society. Lesbians were also just plain worse off economically
than gay men: consequently their interests, alliances, and culture reflected this
difference. White gay male culture—except for those segments affected by alternative philosophies such as the Radical Fairies and the Gay Liberation
Front—was primarily a celebration of male and gay culture without the radical-
izing addition of feminism.[16]

A major distinction between lesbians and gay men, as articulated in publications and politics of the seventies, was in their differing notions of what sexual
freedom meant. Models of sexuality for lesbians that dominated the seventies
were a result of women's socialization and feminism. There are those who say it's
nature and those who say the cause is oppression,[17] but most of us would agree
that almost all women, including lesbians, have been strongly affected by a pattern of socialization that emphasizes the importance of relationships, networks,
care-giving and nurturance.[18] Even though lesbians may have a demonstrated

ability to resist certain aspects of female socialization (males as sexual-object choices, for example), they are not immune to these cultural pressures.

Common wisdom in lesbian culture of the late seventies and early eighties asserted that lesbians form couples and model their dyads on romantic love and enduring relationships. This popular notion was complemented and perhaps strengthened by research on "fusion" in lesbian relationships that emphasized the tendency to blur boundaries between self and other, and identified female socialization as a source of this tendency.[19] A second pervasive aspect of female socialization has been the historical and contemporary emphasis on monogamy, tied partly to patriarchal possessiveness, but also to the risk of pregnancy and the need for legitimate paternity.

In contrast to these two aspects of female socialization, male socialization has emphasized individuation and non-monogamy. While gay men, like lesbians, challenge traditional sex roles, they are, similarly and simultaneously, drawn to them. Gay male sexuality in the seventies was marked by the conflation of sexual experimentation, freedom, and individuality. Gay male and lesbian sexualities and the value systems associated with them were important sources of separation between men and women within the homosexual community during the 1970s.

The message of gay liberation for men was one of self-expression that celebrated male socialization. This meant multiple partners, self-assertion, and "individuation," i.e., experimentation. Gay male sexuality had involved multiple sex partners before gay liberation; the gay movement basically legitimized gay life "as it was." In the early seventies, there were some voices of gay male liberation that provided a critique of traditional male sexuality, including the suggestion that gay men might form their own families, whether of a communal type or more "nuclear" versions. By the end of the decade, more gay men had created families (in some cases linked to lesbians) that included children. However, as the gay movement became institutionalized, it lost much of its radical critique of sexism. There was no movement comparable to feminism to effectively challenge male socialization.

The seventies saw a rapid increase in public gay male culture, institutions, and political influence (including the first candidate, Harvey Milk, to be elected on a gay rights platform). Within these new institutions, struggles over the appropriate nature of gay male life appeared. Writers began to speak of "gay identity" and "community" replacing "homosexual behavior" and "populations." While gay men were in some cases able to claim actual locations for their community centers—the Castro in San Francisco, Greenwich Village in New York—lesbians existed more as a relational or fictional community, often on the geographical fringe of gay men's areas, but usually spread more widely and less distinct as a community.

While lesbians were especially connected to the feminist community and institutions, it seems that gay men were more connected to dominant social institutions. Thus, when the seventies ended and the AIDS epidemic exploded, most lesbians and gay men were living essentially parallel lives, organized primarily around the separate themes of female values and feminism for the women and masculinity and justice for the men.

When the epidemic emerged in the early 1980s, women were immediately affected. They were present as caretakers, educators, physicians, public health officials, community activists and patients. As a diverse social group linked by gender in an epidemic where gender and sexuality are key, women, and lesbians in particular, played powerful symbolic, sexual, and social roles.

The basic arenas of AIDS activity might usefully be sorted into five institutional foci: medical (including research), public health, educational, caring services, and political. In 1980, women in the U.S. (including lesbians) were occupationally placed in large numbers where they would be likely to encounter men with HIV. In medical settings they comprised most of the nursing staff as well as a significant proportion of nurses' aides, home health workers, medical clerical staff, and an increasing number of physicians. Women also dominated the frontline work force in social work and therapy. They were well represented in public health, especially in health education. Within the lesbian and gay community, because women outnumber men in the helping professions, many of the service organizations that were co-sexual had numerous female staff.

These professional roles, whether in straight or gay institutions, draw on traditional nurturing and service models for female activity. But while some lesbians may have been completely traditional in their attitudes toward their work, most had been recently affected by the enormous changes in lesbian culture and institutions that occurred in the 1970s.

Though there are many lesbian perspectives on AIDS, there are four that have dominated. The first view is that lesbians make a distinctive contribution to the struggle. The second approach emphasizes the need for equal funding and services. The third emphasis is on the importance of coalition-building concerning the epidemic, especially the need for coalitions between lesbians and gay men. The fourth analysis is that lesbians should separate themselves from men's concerns vis à vis the epidemic and focus on their own needs, either in terms of HIV issues or their needs in other areas.[20] These perspectives have developed somewhat chronologically during the course of the epidemic as women have increasingly participated in various institutional and movement responses.[21]

The Distinctive Contribution of Women

"AIDS needs women's help," it has been said. This approach characterized the first few years of the epidemic, and was and continues to be most commonly expressed by women working in health care and human services.

Women who take this approach argue that they have special skills to bring to the AIDS response and that as women and lesbians, we have an obligation to share them with our gay brothers. What do women bring? Compassion; experience in the women's health movement, health care skills, nurturing skills; experience with illness; ability to express emotions; relational abilities for organizational growth and change. In fact, many lesbians did bring these skills and styles with them to their work in AIDS. The dominant AIDS organizations for the first half of the decade (1981-86) were health care, service, and education organizations. Initially, most of the clients were men. Within these organizations, lesbians played a variety of nurturing and relational roles. In some cases, women acted as leaders. In most cases, their contribution was underreported and underrated.

The Women's AIDS Network, located in the San Francisco Bay Area, was founded by a mixed group of lesbians and straight women in 1982 at an early national AIDS conference. Overwhelmingly, members of the organization, led primarily by lesbians, were highly educated AIDS professionals:[22] nurses, doctors, therapists, and health educators. Similar to the women in Melissa McNeill's 1991 study of nineteen prominent lesbian AIDS activists,[23] almost all WAN members had prior experience in the feminist movement, health organizing, and/or lesbian and gay civil rights work.

The members of WAN began by giving all they could from what they knew. Giving all you can is not necessarily a feminist activity. In fact, some of the lesbians who worked at the San Francisco AIDS Foundation, as either staff or volunteers, are most appropriately described as non-feminists; some disliked feminism, which they perceived as hostile to gay men (because feminism criticized the men for camp or sexual promiscuousness) or opposed to individual success. Their involvement was more often a result of personal connections with gay men, and less a result of a political analysis. These women were sometimes unsympathetic to their more feminist co-workers, especially when they presented feminist agendas concerning services for women. They interpreted such behavior as uncaring of men.[24]

Most of the lesbians who got involved in AIDS research, service, and policy work in the early years, however, were both feminists *and* nurturers who saw themselves connected politically and ethically to the various populations at risk for AIDS.

The idea that women have special nurturing skills has frequently been expressed and appreciated in AIDS organizations, including those dominated by men. But the special skills associated with women's organizational experience were less acknowledged. This finding held true in McNeill's study as well as in my own research and experience in San Francisco.[25]

Equal Rights for Women/Lesbians in the AIDS World

Soon after women became engaged in the work of the epidemic, a second perspective began to be expressed: that women, as AIDS workers and as people at risk for AIDS, are the victims of sexism and secondary status within the AIDS movement.

Equal rights advocates hold that we need to examine every strategic response to the epidemic to make certain that women's and lesbians' unique needs are met and that there is no potential for oppression or exploitation. Tara's impassioned plea for services for lesbians with HIV is squarely in this tradition. Reproductive rights, civil liberties, motherhood and maternal transmission, the scapegoating of prostitutes, equal access for women—and children—to AIDS education, treatment, social services, food banks, and so on: these issues were all addressed by lesbians and straight women alike. They saw the equal rights approach as necessary because most AIDS policy was determined by and for men, whether by community-based organizations or governmental agencies.

I was privy to one example of this kind of sexism when I worked at the San Francisco AIDS Foundation in the mid-1980s. At the time, I was coordinator of the women's program and supervisor of the development and distribution of educational materials. I oversaw the development of most of the brochures issued by the Foundation, which were being distributed nationally. The Women's AIDS Network had agreed to work jointly with the Foundation to produce what would be the first brochure written specifically for lesbians. However, when I went to my supervisor, a gay man who was director of the education department, to get his formal approval before printing, I was turned down for the first time in my work at the Foundation. I was told that my brochure would not be approved for printing because "lesbians are not at risk for AIDS." Needless to say, within a week, WAN was using its contacts within and without the organization to reverse the decision and eventually (after three months of lobbying) the brochure was published. The director rationalized his about-face: "Well, lesbians aren't really at risk, but since they are working so hard in AIDS services, they deserve a brochure." Thousands of copies were sold and distributed within the first year. The conflict revealed how invisible lesbians were as women at risk, as activists, and as experts in 1985.

In North American AIDS work, championing the equal rights focus for women often means emphasizing class and race, because most women with HIV are poor and either of African American or Latina descent. Lesbians, who have been the primary representatives of straight women as well as themselves, often walked a fine line when they spoke about their own needs for visibility. What did it mean to speak for "women" if one were also lesbian? As the international demographic and epidemiological facts have hit home (although slowly) in the U.S., heterosexual women received consistently more attention, but lesbians lagged far behind. Formal definitions of risk categories for HIV continued to reflect lesbian invisibility. For example, in 1992, the Centers for Disease Control still excluded any woman from its "lesbian" sexual risk category if she'd had sex with a man even once since 1977.

Both the "equal rights" and the "distinctive contribution" approaches to AIDS emerged most strongly during the first half of the first decade of AIDS. By 1987, many AIDS organizations were beginning to react more angrily to the stress of inadequate funding. Additionally, the dream of quick medical solutions and rapid research advances had faded. As a result, direct action tactics became more popular. ACT-UP and its clones were born and spread rapidly throughout the United States and Europe. Lesbians were active members and strategists in these organizations. Many supported the idea of building coalitions and alliances to fight the epidemic politically.

Lesbians and Gay Men Must Form Coalitions

Coalition lesbians argue that lesbians (and for that matter, everyone) should work on improving AIDS policies (even if the particular policy would primarily benefit men), because ultimately these policies affect communities and populations that include lesbians as well as gay men. AIDS, in this view, is a non-gendered "homosexual" issue and to some an issue for all who are economically or criminally marginalized: the underclass, drug users, prostitutes, poor women, and people of color. Coalitionists argued that many recent civil rights restrictions, justified as necessary because of AIDS, are based on homophobia. Furthermore, they said, the rise in anti-gay violence and the loss of community leaders, friends, and family through illness and death, all affected lesbians as well as gay men. They also argued that focusing on AIDS discrimination was the best strategy for ending discrimination against gay people because the two discriminations (AIDS discrimination and homophobia) were completely enmeshed. Further, there was funding and some political interest in dealing with AIDS discrimination.[26]

Many women AIDS activists who shared the coalition perspective also viewed the AIDS epidemic as an opportunity to move toward such broader social agendas as national health care, local housing and shelters, or effective and humane drug policy. They saw these changes as key to improving the role of women, gay people, and many other marginalized groups.

This approach to AIDS work is often associated with an activist stance. McNeill found that of the half of her sample group who were primarily involved in ACT-UP and OUT! (the Washington, D.C. version of ACT-UP), the major appeal was social change. Many stated positions which indicated that they saw AIDS work as a way of approaching the broader society and making changes in it. In my own interviews with lesbian members of ACT-UP in New York, all stated that they saw their work as part of coalition politics. All were feminists who defined themselves as sex radicals.

Divisions within the ACT-UP organizations in several cities suggested that the definition of coalition politics varied. While some women supported the narrow definition of lesbians, gay men, and others working together specifically around AIDS (the initial perspective of ACT-UP New York), others were more attuned to the broader critique of society. These women helped form the branches of ACT-UP and other AIDS activist organizations that have emphasized structural aspects of health and health care which go beyond AIDS treatment per se.

It is partly out of the bonds created between lesbian and gay male AIDS activists, symbolized in organizations like ACT-UP, that Queer Nation, gay anti-violence patrols, and queer cultural institutions were formed. These new, explicitly multi-cultural groups, in which women fill many leadership roles, speak primarily with the voices of the second generation after Stonewall; many of these women and men came of age during the eighties. However, here, too, the legacies of racism and sexism have not been overcome. These organizations continue to break apart over challenges to the maintenance of a white male model of power.

Separatist Approach

While coalition work was expanding within the lesbian community, a previously traveled route was being explored by the "older generation" of lesbians—withdrawal and separatism. Separatist lesbians argue that both feminist and lesbian health priorities should not be focused on AIDS but on other, worse problems affecting women. For example, breast cancer strikes and kills many more women than does AIDS.[27] Gender-related poverty and powerlessness are seen by these activists as more serious health hazards than HIV disease. Separatists argue that women suffer from the current AIDS funding and organizing focus because across the board there is less money and attention paid to women's health issues.[28]

Additionally, some lesbians argue that even if they themselves see AIDS as a major threat to their political and social communities, this is not the way the average person feels in communities that are not primarily gay-identified—African Americans, Latinos, homeless people, poor whites. Therefore AIDS-focused organizing is not an effective way to move toward organizing these communities, including their lesbian members, for survival. A reverse perspective on this argument is that for African American women, AIDS is more of a threat than a "women's illness" like breast cancer because HIV disease is the number one cause of death for both African American women and men in their reproductive years.

While some lesbians may have stayed "out of AIDS" from the beginning because they were unconnected to gay men, did not see themselves at risk, or just wanted to avoid the whole thing, many who were engaged have left full-time AIDS-related work, some to work in other areas and others to do part-time volunteer activity. Of McNeill's subjects, despite their early leadership roles, one in four had turned their attention elsewhere by 1991. Three-quarters were working primarily on women's AIDS issues and other health matters specifically affecting women and lesbians.[29]

No matter what size or type of AIDS organization one examines, these four perspectives appear among lesbians. In the more radical activist organizations, like ACT-UP, we are more likely to find the coalitionists, but during a three-month visit with New York ACT-UP in 1989, I found that the "distinctive contribution" idea was one of the strongest motivators for highly political women. Their distinctive contribution happened to be their organizing skills gained in other direct action and civil disobedience movements. Consistently, these skills were derived from experience with feminist organizing innovations—consciousness raising, affinity groups, and other techniques to assure participatory democracy.

There is no one predominant lesbian (or female) perspective on AIDS. Even within fairly cohesive AIDS organizations with explicit values and priorities concerning the epidemic and women, there is considerable variation. The priorities of women who have been active in AIDS organizations have undergone considerable change as the organizations themselves grew—and shrank—and as the nature of the epidemic, and the federal, state, and local responses to it have changed. We should expect these transformations in priorities to continue.

In addition to political and philosophical differences among lesbians concerning AIDS work, there are also generational differences. Of those lesbians who got involved in the AIDS epidemic in the first five years, some have stayed in the field and have become career AIDS professionals. Others have moved into allied fields (health education, public health, systems management), in some cases with a focus on women. A third group has left AIDS and health altogether, an option that as far as I can tell, is being pursued primarily by those women who were more tangentially engaged, either because of a single friendship or because it was a job.

While some lesbians have been able to become AIDS professionals and remain confrontational activists, this does not seem to be common. McNeill found considerable hostility between the professionals and the activists in her sample. The professionals referred to the activists as irresponsible and ill-informed, while some of the activists thought that the professional women were co-opted. I believe that while there may have been the traditional hostility between members of the movement and the institutionalized service sector, there is also a generational split, reflecting major societal change in the last twenty years and its impact on these groups.

The differences between the older lesbians and the younger generation are deep, widespread in the lesbian community, and in many cases quite antagonistic. They affect how and why lesbians do or do not do AIDS work. They also affect how lesbians not involved with AIDS view the epidemic, safe sex, and lesbians who are connected to HIV and AIDS issues. Although the epidemic itself has helped to shape these differences, other social, economic, and cultural factors have also been at work.

Lesbians who are today predominantly in their thirties and forties grew up in the sixties and were influenced both by more traditional female socialization and by the radical activism of the civil rights movement, anti-war demonstrations, and nascent feminism. In the seventies, when many came of age and came out, feminism was strong and the opportunity to be "out" relatively easily as a lesbian was new. For many of these women simply "being" a lesbian and being public about it was a revolutionary sexual step.

The next generation, on the other hand, came of age and came out in the eighties—a decade marked by explicit debates about sexuality, much greater openness about what would have been called deviant behavior ten years earlier, and broad female access to education. The 1980s were also a time of deepening economic depression and growing radicalism among gay men, as the epidemic remained "uncured" and the failed health economy slammed into their lives. The younger generation of lesbians has less faith in education and government, less of a sense of individual futures, and their sexual radicalness goes beyond being a lesbian. Being able to be a lesbian is more of a given than it was even ten years ago, and for many lesbians of the current generation it is a very limiting identity.

During the eighties, gay men explored safe sex and brought everything from fisting, dildoes, and rimming to nipple rings, golden showers, and sado-masochistic scenes into public discussion, especially within the gay community. This discussion was audible and visible, carried on in a gay press read by both men and women. Increasingly, lesbians, and especially the younger ones, sought access to this world of experimentation. Sexual activity that goes far beyond feminist notions of equality and non-violence became exciting options to the new generation. While some older feminist lesbians looked on in disappointment, younger women (and a few of their older friends) attended bars named Faster Pussycat or the G-Spot, and sex clubs like the Ecstasy Lounge, where cruising, S/M, public sex, and such skills as the safe use of dildoes were being (re)introduced to a new generation.

The younger generation of lesbian AIDS activists carries a different psychology, culture, politics, and sexuality from those who came to the movement in the early eighties. These activists are connected to the older women by the term "lesbian" and by some similarities of sexual practice. Many, however, see their elders as sexually repressed, conservative, and somewhat anti-male.

The two groups may be separated by certain common sources of cross-generational conflict (the inevitable activist mellowing that comes with age and the fact that the older women could be—and in some cases are—the parents of the younger women). But it is the social changes of the eighties that have provided a different sexual and political framework and have led to a new sexuality and its political expression. The new sexuality includes an ever more pointed critique of sexual identities and practices that are organized through the dichotomous categories of *male* and *female*. That sexuality is part of a more radical approach to HIV as well. It's practitioners are more likely to support needle exchange, harm reduction theory,[30] and tolerance of many types of sexual expression, drug use, and risk.

These views of women and AIDS—two first-person accounts of illness and struggle, a policy justification, a radical view, and a sociological analysis of lesbian activism—provide some divergent female perspectives on the epidemic. They vary in emotional force, style, political perspective, and causal argument. But they agree that the voices of women were not heard in the halls of AIDS policy-making and implementation during the eighties and that women's invisibility and powerlessness led to unnecessary deaths. They also agree that the only way to reduce this exclusion is for women to speak and act collectively.

The organizations profiled in the next four chapters were invented out of a similar desire: to save the lives of people who have been ignored or consigned to illness or death in the face of the epidemic. Just as the women in this chapter spoke from a variety of locations which affected their perspectives and analyses, so the organizations profiled represent the diverse life situations and world views of their members. These dissimilarities have led to radically different organizational approaches to the epidemic. In some cases the work of one organization may even harm the population served by another. How this can be and what we might do about it are the subjects of the rest of this book.

Going Mainstream:
The San Francisco AIDS
Foundation

The San Francisco AIDS Foundation (SFAF) began in 1982 as a small, all-volunteer, grassroots activist, educational, and service organization. Fifteen years later it was a stable and dominant force in AIDS prevention and policy. The organization's history provides an example of a white, male, gay-run and gay-focused, politically moderate response to the epidemic. It also represents an archetypal, and often envied pattern of movement from a grassroots volunteer organization to a multimillion-dollar-a-year bureaucracy. Its developmental problems are similar to those faced by other AIDS organizations that were founded and developed by predominantly white male activists. For these reasons, its solutions to structural conflict can clarify processes that other expanding bureaucracies experience.

The Foundation's organizational history, detailed below, also helps explain San Francisco AIDS politics and provides a background to four other organizational developments described in this book. Partly as a response to the limitations of the Foundation's prevention programs, the city witnessed the emergence of a variety of ethnic-based AIDS organizations, including those based in Asian and Pacific Islander communities (Chapter 3). Both Cal-PEP's street outreach (Chapter 4) and Prevention Point's needle exchange (Chapter 5) received Foundation support. The last organization studied in depth, NYC ACT-UP, was born on the opposite side of the continent (Chapter 6), but its raison d'être was to provide an alternative to community-based AIDS bureaucracies, particularly the Gay Men's Health Crisis, which as an organization was very similar to the SFAF in its leadership philosophy, structure, and size. I also selected the AIDS Foundation, Cal-PEP, Prevention Point, and ACT-UP for comparison because each has chosen a very different organizational mode.

Much has been written about the struggles of AIDS organizations to combat forces of external repression, especially in regard to explicit references to sexuality in AIDS education and saving the lives of injection drug users. But little analysis has been done of attempts by AIDS organizations to overcome the internally damaging effects of institutionalized systems of racism, sexism, heirarchy, and stigma. After describing the Foundation's growth process, I examine the ways its leaders dealt with three difficult challenges: serving women, incorporating racial specificity in its safe sex campaigns, and sharing its resources with ethnic communities.

At the beginning of the AIDS epidemic in the United States, disbelief and horror spread through the white gay community as the realization that AIDS was a real and transmissible illness gradually reached the gay community's members and leaders and permeated the networks of straight and gay professionals who worked with gay men with HIV. Shock, denial, and anger were predominant responses to the realization that so many were dying and were going to die. How could it happen? Even when people knew it and had to believe it was true, and therefore did believe it rationally, many could not accept it emotionally. The horror of the epidemic meant the failure of systems they had believed in: modern medicine, individual success, white and male privilege, American privilege. Those who did not succumb to AIDS, depression, internalization, or the overwhelming amount of work necessary to survive with dignity and some measure of happiness developed a more radical and activist perspective, as well as an increasingly national focus. This oppositional approach already was widespread in the African American, Latino, Asian, and Native American communities which have traditionally been excluded and, because they experienced the hard truths of racism, have generally been freer of deep illusions about national compassion.

Cleve Jones' story, told at the National Skills Building Conference in 1995, summarizes these transitions. Jones, a white gay activist and founder of the Names Project, was one of the early activists who began the organizing that resulted in the birth of the San Francisco AIDS Foundation.

I got involved in 1980-81. I saw the newspaper articles about pneumocystis and KS [Kaposi's Sarcoma]. I had been an activist in the gay liberation movement and had worked with Harvey Milk. After his assassination, I became the beneficiary of probably what was the first gay patronage in California politics. I was hired by the Speaker of the [California State] Assembly to be a consultant working on health issues. It was in that capacity that I received a call from Dr. Marcus Conant asking to sit down and meet with me. He took me out to dinner at the Zuni Cafe on Market Street and told me about a young man that he was taking care of named Simon Guzman, a Mexican American man who was very close to death at that point. Marcus did not have any concrete evidence at that time but he told me—and those of you who have heard his presentations or who know him, know that he is a very forceful person—and he said to me then that he thought it would prove to be a virus, that it would be sexually transmitted, and probably the best model we could look at would be hepatitis.

Shortly after that dinner he took me up to meet this young man Simon, and it broke my heart because he had a photograph of himself on the table next to his bed. It showed this beautiful, strong, vibrant young Latino man in Speedos, and I looked at his devastated body just covered with lesions. He died about three days later.

The following week I was walking down Castro Street, and my friend Hank Wilson called me into one of the bars. He was sitting there with a young man named Bobby

Campbell. Bobby was a nurse and a member of the Sisters of Perpetual Indulgence.[1] Bobby took off his shoes and showed me these spots on the bottom of his feet. They were the same spots that had covered Simon's body. I can't remember what his original name was with the Sisters of Perpetual Indulgence but after his diagnosis he became Sister Florence Nightmare.

To me my activism was a natural outgrowth of my work in gay liberation, and the early days were very much grassroots, ad hoc. Most of us did not have degrees. We were just gay activists who were trying to alert our brothers. It was terribly frustrating. I remember when Bill Kraus and I co-authored an article that was printed in the Bay Area Reporter before there were any other articles in the gay papers. We said our take on it was, let's just assume it's like hepatitis. That is a safe assumption. Let us look at precautions as if it were hepatitis. So we talked about multiple partners. We talked about anal sex, and the reaction was unbelievable.

I had people spit on me on Castro Street. I had people call me a Nazi, a sexual fascist. I thought of myself as a sexual liberationist. It was so disheartening.

A lot has changed since then. One of the most significant transitions was the shift from grassroots, ad hoc organizing to institutionalized career options, the bureaucracy. We are all a part of it. It was hard for me to accept, and it becomes harder for me to accept as the years go along.

I've been very lucky. I didn't get sick until April, but I'm not doing very well, and I have to say I have never felt such bitterness and such despair that, with all of our work and all of the suffering and death and pain that we have endured, that we continue to fail. And in my city the infection rates among young gay men are soaring. We have failed. And now I see the third President in a row who will not lead, who will not act, who does not care, and who has done absolutely nothing.

I was talking with my friend Bob Hathcoate [Clinton's advisor]—we have a long history together and I love him very much. I said to him, "Bob, you know I've had all sorts of opportunities to speak. I've stood at all sorts of podiums. I have spoken to thousands and thousands of people, and at this point I don't know what to do. I don't know what to say, but I am very, very frightened."

I know that many of you are also infected, and many of you are also sick. I do not want to die. I do not want to be written off. I want them to find a cure. I want the President and the Congress to move. That's all I can say.[2]

The first San Francisco education and referral organization specifically focused on gay men and AIDS was established in April 1982, after reports of gay men dying from Kaposi's Sarcoma had spread through the Castro area of San Francisco at an alarming rate. Its primary street staff by the end of the year consisted of two volunteers. They collected donations on Castro Street, the major gay thoroughfare, produced informational flyers, and set up a phone line with the beginnings of a referral system. The organization called itself the Kaposi's Sarcoma Foundation, taking its name from the most striking of the diseases associated with the deadly epidemic and using the term "foundation" as a way of encouraging donations.

This was the birth of what was to become the San Francisco AIDS Foundation. For the first six years of the epidemic it was the only organization in San

Francisco to receive public funding for education. It is still one of the major AIDS organizations in the U.S.

The story of the AIDS Foundation is one of incredible achievement, in which an ever-changing group of men and women borrowed from public health, marketing, community organizing, corporate management, social work, and gay cultural traditions to create an organized institutional response to the epidemic. Despite some stumbling and disorganization in the first few years, in part because many volunteer workers were battling illnesses due to HIV infection, these activists and their organizational descendents created a multimillion dollar non-profit bureaucracy.

SFAF received its first contract from the San Francisco Department of Public Health in October 1982, to provide education and an information and referral service. The service became the Northern California AIDS Hotline in 1983, when the agency expanded its contracts to include the State of California Department of Health Services, which provided funds for toll-free access. Direct services to people with AIDS or ARC (as HIV disease was then called) were begun as well, staffed by volunteers.

By early 1984, there were ten staff members, all gay or lesbian. By the next spring, there were twenty-two, two of whom were people of color[3] and all of whom were gay, lesbian, or bisexual. The organization changed its name from the KS Foundation to the KS/AIDS Foundation and, finally, in late 1984, simply to the San Francisco AIDS Foundation. By then it had incorporated and was in its second year of city and state funding.

Initially, the AIDS Foundation served the wealthy and the middle class, as well as the poor, because HIV infection occured among people of all economic strata who were linked by accidental encounters with an unknown virus. In its second decade, as the wealthy learned how to avoid it, AIDS would become more of a class-linked disease, but in the early 1980s class was no protection. In addition, once infected, the carriers knew no escape from illness and death, regardless of class background. Money provided no cures. Therefore, attracting wealthy supporters (especially gay men) as donors, board members, volunteers, and even staff was not difficult. Wealthy donors were less available to AIDS agencies that worked explicitly with the poor and in social and ethnic communities that lacked access to a strong financial base—women, ethnic minorities, rural groups, and drug users seeking safe needles.

As the staff of SFAF increased in size, the necessity for bureaucratic management grew. Charismatic leadership, which produces work by organization members because they believe in and are inspired by their leader, became less useful and a potential hindrance. San Francisco's Shanti Project, which provided direct care to people with AIDS, held on to its initial charismatic leader, Jim Geary, for years, through considerable growth. When Geary finally quit, it was under a cloud of accusations about mismanagement.[4] The San Francisco AIDS Foundation, on the other hand, went through four executive directors and two acting directors while the organization grew from three to eighty-five employees over a period of five years.[5] This may have made for a better match between leadership and organizational needs, because the complexity of a bureaucratic organization requires a variety of management skills and the stabilization that comes from clear roles and responsibilities. These aspects of growth are further discussed in Chapter 7. The AIDS Foundation's annual reports provide a means to look at the agency's changing self-presentation, programmatic priorities, board composition, and budget. These reports also document the agency's transition from grass roots community organization to multi-million dollar non-profit. To review the history of the organization, I draw on the reports, internal documents, materials used in public education campaigns, field notes, interviews with staff, public comments by current and former members, and press coverage.

In 1984, the San Francisco Department of Public Health began funding the social services of the agency, and by April a client services department of three social workers and an administrative assistant was serving 150 clients. In the Foundation's 1985 *Annual Report*,[6] Bob Bolan, the president of the board of directors, began his official message with an explicit commitment to bureaucratic growth, internal efficiency, and professionalism:

> As we mark the passage of another year in the AIDS epidemic we must realize that while we remain hopeful that its horrible secrets will be unlocked and that its devastation will be stopped, we must prepare for a very long siege. For the San Francisco AIDS Foundation that means striving to become an ever more efficient, thoroughly professional agency. We must compete for charitable donations alongside many other similar, non-AIDS agencies with comparably noble missions; we must achieve and maintain impeccable management skills, political and fiscal savvy so that we can influence governmental funding for AIDS education and social services. In short, we must continue to hope that the epidemic will be contained within the near future. But we must plan and act as though we are building a responsive agency that must continue its mission well into the next century. We are honored and humbled to play such a vital role in the community's response to this awful disease.[6]

That same year the agency's budget passed the million dollar mark, a step that foreshadowed its continued growth over the next decade. Approximately $885,000 of the 1985 income was from public grants. The agency also raised $123,000 in organizational donations, $179,000 from individuals, and $41,000 from a benefit. Although a substantial portion of the agency's income (72 percent) was from governmental sources, this was already a better mix of private funds than many non-profits are able to maintain. A continuing source of the Foundation's economic strength was its ability to tap large pockets of cash because it had access to well-connected fund raisers, corporations, and individuals with inherited wealth or high incomes.

In 1985, the Foundation still held the only San Francisco Department of Health contract for educational services, which it had first obtained in 1983. It provided speakers, sponsored trainings, generated and distributed materials, and worked with the media. Its primary focus was on gay and bisexual men, "the groups at highest risk in San Francisco."[7] Its state-funded programs for the hotline and its Northern California outreach continued. In that year the agency also began a conscious expansion of its educational outreach to ethnic minorities, women at risk, intravenous drug users, heterosexuals at risk, and prison inmates. External pressures to shift funding from SFAF to other community organizations with stronger roots in communities of color were just beginning to intensify. They reached the breaking point in 1986 and resulted in new funding patterns in 1987 that provided the economic base for organizations that are now run by ethnic minorities, such as the California Prevention Education Project.

In 1983 SFAF had secured funding from the state Department of Health Services to provide technical assistance to local groups in Northern California, do some direct education, and run the Northern California AIDS hotline. Through its social services programs, the agency provided counseling and housing. It also ran a Food Bank; in 1985, approximately 110 people a month received food. The other major activity of the Foundation was advocacy for people with AIDS and HIV. This work was largely funded out of private donations, although, like many organizations, SFAF was able to define what some might call advocacy as education or social service and thereby support it with public funding. The death of Rock Hudson in 1986 sparked greater public interest in AIDS and the workload and budget of SFAF grew accordingly. By 1993, the Foundation's budget had reached $7.7 million.

Tim Wolfred, a psychologist and a participant in San Francisco's political and governmental world, was hired as executive director in 1985. With some nonprofit management experience and a term as an elected member of the San Francisco Community College Board of Directors (he later served as its president), Wolfred brought a combination of gay community backing, political legitimacy, and bureaucratic experience to the agency. With the support of the board, and to the relief of most of the staff, which had been both exhilarated and traumatized by rapid growth and multiple management changes, Wolfred moved the agency systematically in the direction of a professionalized bureaucracy. One of Wolfred's innovations was to bring in a management consultant to run a year-long process of organizational analysis, planning, and restructuring to help deal with internal problems that were surfacing as the organization's focus changed from community organizing and self-help to professional service delivery.

These changes from small to large and volunteer to professional staff had several correlates in policy and program development. Most apparent, was the accelerated movement away from confrontation and direct action to a more liberal politics of inclusion in the broader social and economic structure. The San Francisco AIDS Foundation's criticism of an ACT-UP demonstration on the Golden Gate Bridge in 1987 is a perfect example of this change. San Francisco ACT-UP stopped all traffic on the bridge to protest the lack of progress in treatment research and to make the public aware of the frustrations of people with

AIDS. Although SFAF had been founded by community activists, by 1987 its budget was dependent on donations from middle- and upper-class individuals, precisely those who might cross the bridge to work each day from the wealthy suburban towns of Marin County to the north of San Francisco. The Foundation also required good relations with local government agencies. While the staff may have agreed with the concerns of the demonstrators, the Foundation's commitment was to obey the law. Consequently the agency officially criticized the demonstration, saying there are other ways of getting one's point across.

Professionalization had also affected the staff of the organization profoundly. Those who were present from the start found themselves outclassed under the terms of new contracts because they lacked degrees. Others, who had not risen quickly enough, slipped into bureaucratic eddies where they were doomed to low salaries while their more centrally located confreres got higher and higher pay and more and more authority.

Through the consulting process the agency moved firmly into a bureaucratic model in which the boundaries between it and its "community" were more sharply drawn. Hierarchically organized lines of authority were clearer; there were more management positions, and salaries were determined by rank, including increasingly higher salaries for top management. The Foundation was becoming structurally indistinguishable from the majority of large and stabilized social service non-profit organizations.

During this period considerable staff unrest began to surface. One staff meeting in particular revealed a number of unaddressed issues, but prime among them, especially for women and people of color, were issues of diversity. Gay men also felt pain associated with their identities. The following quotations are taken from a summary list of issues recorded at the meeting and printed for all the participants.

> "We are 'working hard' to overcome our gay image."
> "To what extent do we buy in to doing 'all' because we are gay/lesbian/bi, etc.?"
> "Being a minority oriented organization we get messages we're bad. No one cares. Leads to mistrust and burnout. Internalized oppression."
> "Turn on each other."
> "We meet often—reason is mistrust."
> "We are 'sexual minority' oriented, not ethnic oriented."
> "As gay people we learned to bond by alienation—now people repeat this habit inside the organization."
> "'Gay' is not the issue—we all bond by alienation."
> "Distrust, insecurity, fear is a habit brought in from past experience, not necessarily valid."[8]

A staff committee (all gay) of two black men, one white man, and one white woman was selected to make a plan to deal with these issues, which were conceptualized as problems of living with diversity.[9] One of the committee's recommendations was to bring in professional trainers for a series of "Unlearning Racism" workshops, a method developed by Ricky Sherover-Marcuse in the early 1980s and still in wide use.[10] Although the majority of the agency's staff responded favorably to this proposal, the agency did not become a model of racial and sexual diversity and good communication as a result. What happened?

The Unlearning Racism approach is based on an assumption that for progress to be made, the participants must *want* to make changes. Unfortunately, this is not always the case when everyone in a bureaucratically run organization is "required" or expected to participate in a workshop. Some of those who initially attended had little motivation or interest. In addition, some thought the entire process was really only for the "disempowered." Individuals with these opinions were more likely to miss the later meetings. The coordinator/facilitator defined this behavior as psychological resistance, but it was social as well.

As a result of the "revisioning" process, the organization did become somewhat more racially diverse, a women's caucus and a people of color caucus were created to provide input, and those making decisions in any context were formally instructed to think about the impact of their actions on "people of color, women, people with AIDS/ARC, board members, volunteers, and staff members at different hierarchical levels."[11]

Nevertheless the external economic and political forces of competition and minority insurgency placed new demands on the organization, while the internal forces—changing clientele, increased size of the staff, more layers to the bureaucracy—did as well. Despite its goal of diversity, the agency and its administration were objects of external and internal attack in regard to issues of race and gender—for its administrative composition, lack of staff-client match, management-employee relations and reorganization strategies (which resulted in closing the official Women's Program and reducing the independence of the Spanish and Filipino hotlines). These conflicts were repeatedly characterized by the groups experiencing discrimination as cases of power and its abuse, lack of communication, inability to handle diversity properly, and arrogance by those who were—in the specific situation—in power.

In the long run, the facilitated professional intervention did not make any significant organizational changes that were strong enough to end these problems. I believe that this is because the organization changed neither its decisionmaking process, nor its upper level staff composition, nor the basic values of its board.

By 1988, the societal response to the epidemic was beginning to change. There were more organizations and more racial diversity in their composition, and this was beginning to have an impact on both the level of public funding for SFAF programs and the sales of the agency's materials. Government agencies were directly funding minority organizations, and purchasers of materials were also buying more from these organizations or creating their own materials.

Tim Wolfred resigned. He had been the executive director for four years and had brought stability and managed growth into the organization. He was replaced by Pat Christen, a white heterosexual woman, who had served as public policy director for the previous two years. Christen settled in for a long stay and was still the executive director in 1997. She had some background in health and management, but she was hired to work in SFAF's education department beginning in 1986 and then as policy director the following year. She was an articulate, liberal advocate and a highly presentable representative of the organization. She was also known for having good management skills. Her selection as executive director was a sign of the agency's desire for stability, continuity, and a nonthreatening relationship with funders and politicians.

The transition to bureaucracy was now complete, and the organization was ready for a structural holding pattern. Christen presided over the re-organization and temporary shrinkage of the Foundation's scope of services. In 1990 she jettisoned the food bank and the materials marketing divisions. The organization kept its client services, education, and policy programs. It then grew once more.

In 1982 there had been fewer than ten organizations or projects in the Bay Area with a primary focus on AIDS; ten years later there were hundreds. Transitions in patterns of government funding and the proliferation of AIDS organizations serving people of color led to a re-evaluation of focus in the Foundation. In 1990 SFAF proclaimed that its educational campaigns were "directed toward gay and bisexual men, injection drug users and their partners, individuals who are HIV-positive, and others at risk for HIV infection." While the expression "others at risk" could include just about everyone, in fact the priorities were those explicitly enumerated. From then on, phrases referring to sexual and ethnic diversity appeared repeatedly in titles of projects. The first page of the 1992 *Annual Report* (re)writes the history of the organization from the standpoint of ethnicity and diversity:

> From the beginning, the AIDS Foundation has maintained a clear understanding of the need to provide meaningful services to those in greatest need. Gay and bisexual men of all colors, who comprise more than ninety-three percent of the AIDS case load in San Francisco, have always been served proudly by our agency. Injection drug users—whether they are actively using substances or are in recovery—have always been welcome here. Lesbian, bisexual, and heterosexual women and transgender individuals, whether African American, Latina, Asian, Pacific Islander, White, or Native American, are treasured members of our community, deserving of compassionate and respectful service from the AIDS Foundation.[12]

It is unclear whether this framing was intended to respond to critics, to describe previous intent (often criticized by minority organizations as falling short in programmatic accomplishment), or to re-affirm current policy. It does, however, indicate the need of the organization to create a sense of public connection between itself and the diverse communities affected by the epidemic. The programmatic expression of multiculturalism is seen most strongly in 1992 in the titles of the client services department's programs: Gay/Bisexual Men of All Colors, Bilingual/Multicultural Services, Women and Children's Services.

The education department's programs remained focused on risk groups described in terms of behavior (sex with men, drug use) without policy-level titles addressing sexual, gender, or ethnic identities. The public policy/communications department worked on funding for the Ryan White CARE Act, needle exchange, and general advocacy efforts at the state level. In these areas—education and policy—the Foundation continued to see itself as the leading organization within the state of California and, in some cases, as one of the most important national players as well.

In 1993 and 1994, the agency further increased its non-governmental funding base and continued to focus on its now clearly-defined mandates. Its status as an "older" organization and an "established" bureaucracy was confirmed by internal and external events. Some members of the Foundation's staff were even called "HIV-negative AIDS leeches" in the gay press.

Perhaps more telling is that throughout 1993 and 1994, SFAF employees were actively engaged in painful—and to management, shocking—attempts to unionize, highlighting the reality of the distance between employees and management. The unionizing drive succeeded with employees joining a Teamsters' Union local. The transition from a volunteer movement organization to a bureaucracy with management and employees was now complete.

Sexing the Services

SFAF's struggles over issues of race and gender were ones in which I was directly involved as a staff member in the education department from 1984 to 1987. In 1986 the education department, with a staff of five, had established a ranking system to express the values, opinions, and priorities of the department members concerning how our budget should be allocated. Naturally the cultural values of the staff had an impact on this process. For example, at a planning meeting in June 1986, the department decided to divide its resources among programs aimed at those with HIV and at five "at-risk" populations—gay men, heterosexuals, needle users, the general population, and mothers and children. There was no mention of programs for specific ethnic and cultural groups. Nor were there any references to women or lesbians. The assumption was that "women" were incorporated in heterosexual transmission prevention work and in materials that identified them as the potential source of HIV in maternal-child transmission. Despite this seeming invisibility, however, the Foundation had an ongoing set of services and materials carved out of other programs by feminists within the agency. But, as the history of these programs indicates, their provision was not without obstacles.

The Foundation had established its first funded program for women in 1984 with a state grant to conduct a needs assessment addressing women and AIDS in Northern California. The grant came to the Foundation—as opposed to the Women's AIDS Network, which also applied for it—because of the state's desire to stick with its primary San Francisco agencies (Shanti and SFAF) for channeling funds. As a compromise, SFAF hired WAN's grant writer, myself, to run the assessment.

The grant covered a six-month period, beginning in December 1984, in which to survey eight counties in Northern California to assess the level of need and existing resources for women in terms of the epidemic. At the end of the grant period, the Foundation retained me by transferring my salary to city grants with primary responsibility for developing and distributing educational materials. My first major project was to act as liaison and technical consultant for a grant to develop materials to accompany the San Francisco introduction of the HIV antibody test.

I was allowed to keep my informal title of women's resources coordinator and my role as advocate for women's services and education both within the Foundation and when working with other agencies. Both to others and to myself, I defined my feminist work as part of my bureaucratic responsibility for development and distribution of educational materials. For example, I saw the preparation of a brochure for women to be part of my wider responsibility to develop brochures. I defined my role as coordinator of the Women's AIDS Network as part of my assignment to foster education and develop resources for women (part of the general mission of the Foundation). With other women at the Foundation and the support of women advocates throughout the AIDS community, we referred to my activities as the "Women's Program," and to myself as its coordinator. Thus the program was invented and continued throughout my time at the Foundation.

Women's calls to the SFAF hotline demonstrated a strong and growing interest in HIV transmission.[13] Several women callers and volunteers at the Foundation complained that they could not find appropriate services for themselves; these were usually women who had had male partners who had died from HIV infection. Some knew they were uninfected; others were unsure. They were uncomfortable in officially mixed support groups in which they generally found themselves to be the only female and the only heterosexual. In addition, none of the callers were drug users, so they felt equally out of place at sessions for drug users or ex-users. In response to these requests, and with some excitement about finding a real need for women's services, SFAF organized an initial meeting with several at-risk women and the staffs of the Foundation and the AIDS Health Project (AHP) run by the University of California at San Francisco. At a later meeting an agreement for a facilitated women's support group at AHP and a non-facilitated group at SFAF was finalized, and the groups began the next month.[14] Despite a slow start at both agencies, these groups led to ongoing direct services specifically for women at these and other San Francisco agencies. AHP continued to provide facilitated short-term (six-week) groups, and SFAF eventually developed a weekly daytime women's drop-in group that operated out of its social services department under the direction and protection of Catherine Maier. By April 1985 fourteen services for women at six agencies had been established.[15]

Because women "at risk of AIDS"[16] fell into several very distinct social group-ings, the Foundation's Women's Program was designed to identify the various categories and develop educational, medical, social, and economic services that met the specific needs of different groups. The needs assessment began this process, which then continued through the use of SFAF, WAN, and other resources. Since women at risk of infection were most likely to be women of color, the program had a multi-racial focus from the start. My own interests in multi-racial, multi-ethnic advocacy affected the women's service projects as well as the educational materials work. In addition, like other staff, I knew I was involved in historic events. I wanted to be proud of my role and to make a difference for those who were being excluded.

A survey of residential drug treatment programs that accepted women revealed that there were no programs that accepted pregnant women or women accompanied by children.[17] The Women's Program wrote to the city's Human Rights Commission; we presented the lack of services as exclusionary and as a human rights issue. We argued that "women's pregnancies and their maternal connections to young children are social and biological aspects of being female."[18] The following year, when the Human Rights Commission held AIDS discrimina-tion hearings, the Women's AIDS Network and the SFAF Women's Program joined together to advocate for greater access for women with AIDS to housing and residential drug programs, with a specific emphasis on the family needs of women. WAN and the Women's Program demonstrated that programs designed to serve individuals—based on a male, white, gay model of individuals separated from their families (through economic emancipation, non-parenting, and/or homophobia)—excluded women *de facto* if not *de jure*.[19] The Program also devel-oped educational materials and events and did advocacy for incarcerated women, prostitutes, women of color, and lesbians.

This work often led to both conflicts and cooperative strategizing with other players in the AIDS world, both within and outside the agency. For example, after being criticized as insensitive to women's needs to find housing with space for children at the Human Rights Commission hearing, the director of Shanti's resi-dential program at first defended her agency, noting that it had been able to take individual women and provide them with housing without any problems. She emphasized that Shanti was 50 percent female in staff. Then, using the hearing testimony as leverage, she initiated a successful process to develop housing for women with children.[20] In this, she was strongly supported by WAN and the SFAF Women's Program.

Two controversies that involved me personally while working at the Foundation demonstrate some of the reasons why problems of sexism and racism are so hard to resolve in an organization run by white men. The first of these encounters, about lesbian visibility, was described earlier (see Chapter 1). The second dealt with race and sexuality, and it emerged in the preparation of a pre-vention brochure prepared for the heterosexual population.

The Color of Sex

When issues of race and gender are combined with discussion or representation of erotic activity, the mix can be explosive. In most AIDS prevention materials, interracial sex is graphically presented as an option for lesbians and gay men. Heterosexuality is usually represented as racially segregated, universally so when families with children are depicted or implied. This distinction is not accidental, but intended, and the San Francisco AIDS Foundation is no exception to the rule.

In 1986 the San Francisco AIDS Foundation began its first campaign to reduce risk of HIV infection among heterosexuals with a grant from the city to conduct focus groups and design a full-scale media campaign to reach heterosexuals at risk. The "focus group" research strategy was in vogue among public health researchers. The strategy, borrowed from advertising and market research, was based on the concept of "social marketing," the idea that social behaviors can be sold, just as products can, and that focus groups can tell educators how to design messages for the public.[21] AIDS Foundation consultant Sam Puckett, with experience in advertising, was a strong advocate of this approach. Together with friends at the city's AIDS Office, he steered SFAF's business to two interlocking San Francisco market research companies run by (white) gay men: Research and Decisions Corporation and Communication Technologies. Since SFAF was at the time the only agency funded by the city to do AIDS prevention research concerning behavioral interventions, its choice of research firms, although approved by the AIDS Office, was basically the final choice. That year, SFAF also delivered its only ethnic outreach research grant to these two firms, which conducted a focus-group study with leaders of African American, Asian, and Latino communities in San Francisco.[22]

On January 24, 1986, Research and Decisions Corporation (R and D) released its focus-group study of sexually active heterosexuals, their perceived risk of HIV infection, and their openness to various messages. This was the fourth study that R and D had done for the city in conjunction with AIDS prevention, the previous three studies being of gay and bisexual men. Utilizing the study results, the education department at SFAF designed an outreach campaign that ultimately became the first bus poster campaign to advocate the use of condoms. Because the campaign was within the scope of heterosexual outreach—my responsibility—I coordinated it, selecting graphics, reserving space, and identifying and resolving political obstacles. Although the large side posters were only up for a month, the bus company in a cooperative gesture left the smaller back posters up as long as possible. I saw the last of them in 1988.

This campaign had two major components: large posters on buses promoting condom use and a brochure with more detailed explanations of risk and protection. In both cases we intentionally developed multi-racial images to reach the varied population of San Francisco.

The bus poster campaign proceeded without difficulties. It presented three couples on bus posters: one African American, one white, and one Latino. In this case, I had argued for human representation so that the individuals seeing the posters would better identify with the messages. There was some opposition among those who had wished to have a graphic that was "neutral" in regard to ethnicity, thereby precluding images of people unless in silhouette. We were able to get a volunteer photographer and free models to produce a variety of visuals that would otherwise have been beyond our budget. The campaign ran from April 1 to May 31, 1987, on buses throughout the city. It was the first public advertising for condom use in San Francisco.

Cost is an often-raised issue in presenting diversified representation: three languages are more expensive than one; multiple graphics cost more money. But when the number of graphics must be limited, there is the question of which graphics to select. When the AIDS Foundation developed its Bleachman campaign, the icon chosen—a cartoon-like, human-size talking bleach bottle—was selected precisely because it could not be identified as having a specific ethnicity, although its gender was inherent in its name. (Should it have been Bleach-person?) The intent there was to avoid privileging (or stigmatizing) one ethnicity over another, as well as to provide a humorous and easily identifiable character to associate with cleaning needles. On the other hand, one could say that Bleachman was the ultimate in white: a white bottle containing a fluid that is symbolically the essence of becoming white. Bleachman is the whitener turned into a living being telling you that not only will bleach make you "white," but it will also save your life. Still, Bleachman was an immediate success in all the neighborhoods he visited. Bleachman literature and comic book spin-offs were also popular, appealing to a variety of English-speaking and low-literacy audiences.

For the heterosexual campaign, bus posters with clear ethnic identities were generated in order to provide explicit role models so that the people seeing them would want to be like the people in the posters: attractive, sexual, and condom-using. (See Illustrations 2.1, 2.2, and 2.3.) Smaller posters on the backs of the buses advertised condoms with text alone. Overall, the bus campaign was deemed a success by the Foundation, generating many hotline calls and receiving additional publicity in the mainstream media.

Things were more complicated with the Foundation's first heterosexual brochure, *Straight Talk about Sex and AIDS.* This brochure was written for an eighth-grade reading level, featured multi-ethnic images, and was printed in English and Spanish. It was published in March 1986. Rock Hudson died later that year. Interest in prevention work with heterosexuals immediately skyrocketed. This interest focused attention on SFAF's heterosexual brochure and, ultimately, on its interracial graphics.

In October 1986, I was surprised to receive a copy of the following memo from Sam Puckett to Jackson Peyton, director of the education department, objecting to the brochure's graphics.

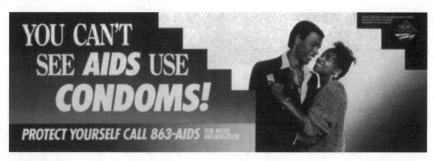

Illustration 2.1

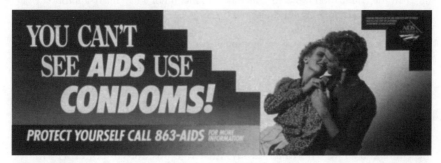

Illustration 2.2

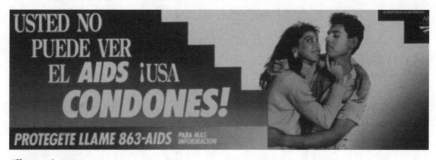

Illustration 2.3

As I indicated, the Mayor is willing to take a leading role in promoting AIDS-prevention for heterosexuals, both locally and nationally. She plans to call a big press conference in December about AIDS and heterosexuals and plans to make a presentation to the Mayor's Conference on the same subject.

She also wants us to develop the "definitive national brochure" for heterosexuals and will promote its use nationally.

"Straight Talk about AIDS" has some limitations. No one seems very excited about it. Amory mentioned that there has been objection to the fact that all the couples pictured are multi-racial. Fawn has mentioned that she's unable to sell the brochure in some states because all the pictures are multi-racial. The multi-racial pictorials were designed to meet the needs of certain local politically-correct audiences, rather than to promote the effectiveness of the brochure. The brochure is also too wordy and too indirect. Amory is convinced the Mayor will not be impressed with it.

If the Foundation wants to undertake production of a nationally-appropriate heterosexual brochure, this is a choice opportunity. The Mayor is a superb salesperson. It could get a lot of publicity.

Maybe this is a job for the marketing department.[23]

Before describing the events that occurred after this memo was distributed, it is useful to identify the characters. Peyton, Puckett, and Amory were all southern, white, gay, and male. Amory was then head of the AIDS Office, Puckett a Foundation consultant, and Peyton the head of the Foundation's education department. These three men were the ones who most wanted to change the brochure and all were bureaucratically situated in positions of power. The Mayor was Dianne Feinstein, known locally for her distaste for gay male sexual promiscuity and known widely for her political ambitions. Fawn was the white, straight female coordinator of materials distribution who filled national and local orders for brochures and other educational materials. "The marketing department" (invented earlier by Fawn and myself) was at this time run by gay men and, prior to that, had been responsible for only one educational project, which was supervised by Puckett. As a result of Puckett's memo, the graphics in the English language version of the brochure were completely redesigned (see Illustrations 2.4 and 2.5) and those in the Spanish format slightly revised.

When looked at closely it becomes clear that this interoffice memo about the inappropriate nature of the graphics expresses an exclusively "white" point of view: A southern state's health director reportedly did not want interracial graphics; no person of color is cited anywhere in the discussion as giving any opinion. The memo indicates that the key blockers of the brochure were Amory and Puckett. Amory had not shown the brochure to the Mayor, but he was sure that she would not like it; he cited objections to the multi-racial couples but did not identify them. Puckett said (inaccurately) that "we have been unable to sell the brochure in some states because all the pictures are multi-racial," and arrogantly commented that the pictures were designed to meet the needs of "certain politically-correct audiences, rather than to promote the effectiveness of the brochure."

Illustration 2.4: *Cover graphics of heterosexual brochure.*

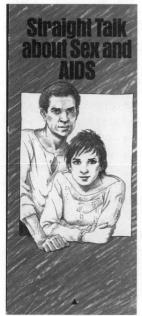

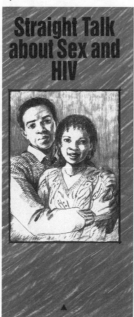

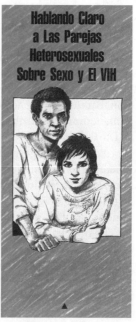

original   *replacement-English*   *retained-Spanish*

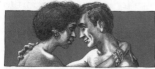

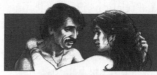

Illustration 2.5: *Interior graphics of heterosexual brochure.*

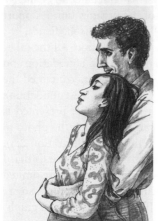

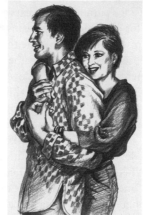

originals   *replacements-English and Spanish*

The first couple in the center brochure, possibly interracial, was replaced by two African Americans in the revised English brochure. There are several visual implications of retaining the "interracial" graphics for the Spanish brochure, as seen on the brochure covers (Illustration 2.4). First, we are being told that people who speak Spanish are not socially segregated by hair type, eye shapes, or skin tone. Simultaneously, by presenting only racially segregated couples for English readers, the authors tell the reader that English speakers are so used to segregation that they would be puzzled by a brochure in which the couples are not racially and ethnically identical. This attitude was further elaborated in a memo from AIDS Office director Amory approving the revision. He commented that the original brochure gave the impression that HIV risk occured only in "situations where sexual partners are from different backgrounds," i.e., different races or ethnicities. Such an idea has never had credence, except perhaps for those who argued that staying away from Haitians and Africans would keep white Americans safe from HIV.[24]

The maintenance of racial order sometimes requires concerted action in the face of change, in this case the presentation of a multiracial brochure. Even liberals have their limits when it comes to race and sexuality, despite their arguments for expanded definitions of sexual expression for themselves. We must also remember that most of the actors in the above scenario were gay men who accepted interracial sex among men and explicit sexual representations in gay educational campaigns.

The original brochure challenged racialized sexual prescriptions of segregation in heterosexual relationships. Projecting their own feelings of discomfort to others, these three men chose to change the graphics and produce a new message. They consciously rearranged the treatment of sex and race to coincide with and reinforce racial segregation. They did not want to challenge racism, only the sexual prudery that was putting heterosexuals at risk. This reluctance to challenge the social order of race parallels other expressions of the organization's support of the legal order, for example, its criticisms of ACT-UP's civil disobedience.

The treatment of the brochure was neither fluke nor aberration. All the other materials for heterosexuals generated by the San Francisco AIDS Foundation and the city's Department of Public Health over the next seven years contained the same racial prescriptions for heterosexual life. For example, in the Foundation's 1994 brochure for straight men about condom use, each couple presented is either white or black, or at least in the same color range, although the photo to the right gives an ambiguous hint of darker skin to the man (Illustration 2.6). This is the closest deviation toward an interracial script for heterosexuals that I was able to find. When the graphics in a heterosexual AIDS brochure are limited to just one image, one sees either a couple of a specific "race" or people who are of some indeterminate ethnicity or racial category (Illustration 2.7). Such graphics may then be used in multiple versions for varying ethnic groups and language communities. Sometimes the only change in the graphics from English to the Spanish version is in the coloring, while the drawing remains the same

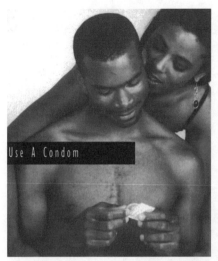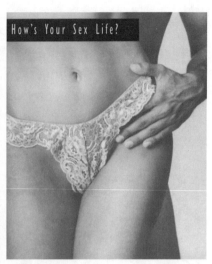

Illustration 2.6: *Safe sex brochure for heterosexual men.*

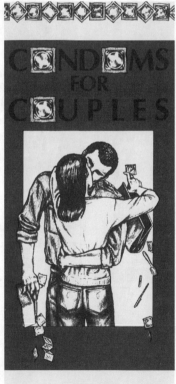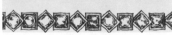

Illustration 2.7:
Condom guide for
heterosexuals.

Illustration 2.8: *Two versions of pregnancy brochure.*

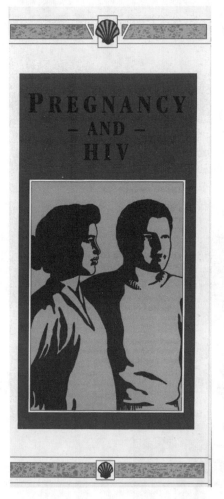
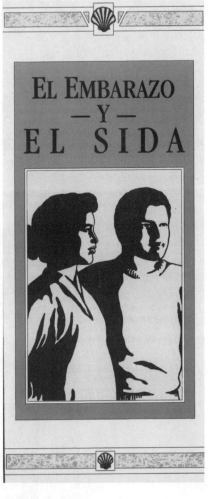

(Illustration 2.8). "Pregnancy and HIV" was printed in peach; "El Embarazo y El Sida" in aqua.

These images project not only racial segregation in AIDS materials, but also the linkage of racial separation and heterosexuality. In contrast to the racial segregation of heterosexuals, many AIDS organizations, including the San Francisco AIDS Office and the San Francisco AIDS Foundation, repeatedly utilize interracial sex scenes and partners when promoting safe sex among gay men. For example, the controversial bus shelter posters of two young men, apparently naked, and wrapped in an American flag, presents a light-skinned blonde and a darker-skinned, dark-haired youth. (see Illustrations 2.9 and 2.10). Lesbians are also presented in interracial sexual relationships (see Illustrations 2.11 and 2.12). A lesbian AIDS graphic from England (Illustration 2.13) is a sample of the international acceptability of interracial sex in the lesbian and gay community and in the world of AIDS prevention—for homosexuals.

On the other hand, the visual message in heterosexual AIDS prevention is racial and ethnic separation. The written and verbal texts focus on reproduction, responsibility, safety, and power. Eroticization is presented primarily as a safety strategy for women, not as a goal in itself. In contrast the texts directed at the gay male audience focus almost exclusively on the eroticization of safe sex, beginning with the idea that sex itself is erotic. Lesbian sexual messages contain a special emphasis on acknowledging and describing risk in order to justify and explain safe sex. In lesbian materials, the erotic is conveyed primarily through the graphics.

Recent race relations theory and cultural analysis have examined the prohibition on heterosexual contact across race lines, as well as the uses of race in the signification of homosexual desire. Writers as diverse as the historian Theodore Allen in *The Invention of the White Race*[25] and the cultural critic Phillip Brian Harper in his "Eloquence and Epitaph"[26] have analyzed the suppression of black male sexuality with regard to both white men and white women.

A key aspect of American racism is the prevention of reproductive mixing, especially between whites and African Americans. Suppression of heterosexual desire across race lines is an important element in the maintenance of the American system of white racialized power. Sex between same-sex partners is, however, less threatening to racial dominance because it is usually viewed as non-reproductive. In addition, same-sex eroticism is fueled by taboo and the forbidden. Since interracial sex is forbidden in the dominant culture and is thus both taboo and exotic, it is often utilized in gay culture both as a spur to sexuality and as a representative or code for erotic encounters.[27] Eroticizing interracial sex does not necessarily mean that gay people are any less racist than heterosexuals, nor does it mean that they consciously reject the valuation of racial purity. Eroticization and valuation of difference are quite compatible with racial stratification.

Why is it so important to examine racial content in AIDS-prevention images? Should we not just subject this discussion to "polite repression," as Toni Morrison says we often do with the topic of race?[28] One reason for not repressing race is that

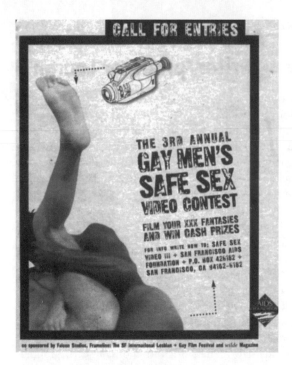

Illustration 2.9: San Francisco AIDS Foundation ad in a gay newspaper, The Bay Area Reporter.

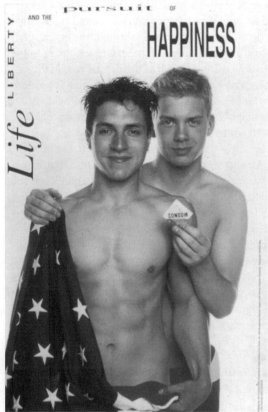

Illustration 2.10: Bus Shelter poster directed at young gay men.

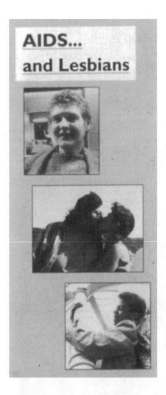

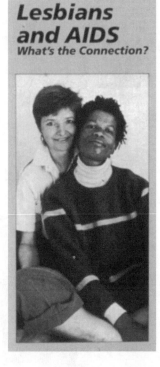

Illustration 2.11:
Safe sex brochures for lesbians from San Francisco AIDS Foundation.

Illustration 2.12: Brochure and stand up cut-out from L.A. Gay & Lesbian Community Services Center.

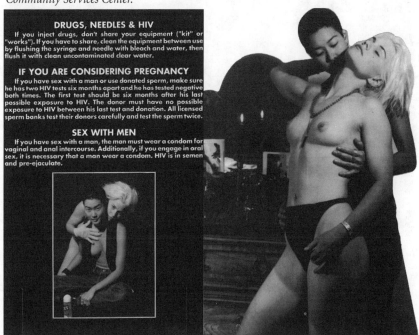

DRUGS, NEEDLES & HIV
If you inject drugs, don't share your equipment ("kit" or "works"). If you have to share, clean the equipment between use by flushing the syringe and needle with bleach and water, then flush it with clean uncontaminated clear water.

IF YOU ARE CONSIDERING PREGNANCY
If you have sex with a man or use donated sperm, make sure he has two HIV tests six months apart and he has tested negative both times. The first test should be six months after his last possible exposure to HIV. The donor must have no possible exposure to HIV between his last test and donation. All licensed sperm banks test their donors carefully and test the sperm twice.

SEX WITH MEN
If you have sex with a man, the man must wear a condom for vaginal and anal intercourse. Additionally, if you engage in oral sex, it is necessary that a man wear a condom. HIV is in semen and pre-ejaculate.

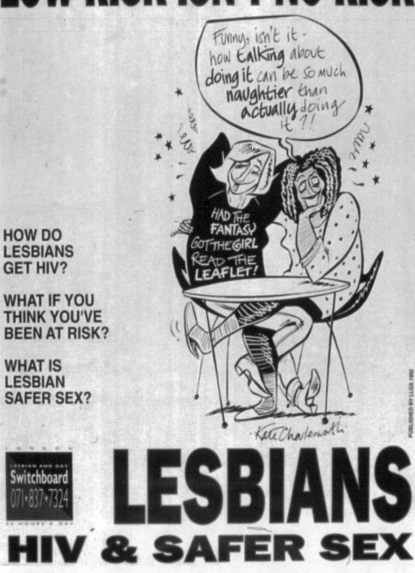

Illustration 2.13: *Poster from Lesbian and Gay Switchboard, London.*

acknowledging and investigating these implicit ideological messages could lead to improvement in the explicit messages contained in AIDS materials. Another reason is that such changes could also modulate the racialized thinking (in particular the categorizing) that is such a key characteristic of American social and political thought.[29] The tendency to racialize and stratify, with the most basic categories being that of white and black, is at the core of American notions of otherness and identity.[30] I would argue that this legacy from chattel slavery sets the stage for our ability to discard those who do not belong to our category and to believe that they are essentially different and less human. This "othering" and devaluation operate powerfully in the abandonment of those with AIDS as well as others who fall into "expendable" categories. So it is in the interest of AIDS activists to address this system of othering, even when it is being expressed in an aspect of community life and education where the activist does not feel immediately engaged. That is, it is in the interest of a gay white man fighting AIDS to become conscious of the role of racial thinking in AIDS-prevention work directed at heterosexuals: because that racism teaches the essentialism and dehumanization of the other which is basic to homophobia and the societal abandonment of homosexuals.

When associations of race and sex are repeatedly reinforced in very powerful sexual materials, the racial and sexual divisions in the U.S. are being reinforced. Being straight and racially segregated is normalized while being gay and integrated is seen as deviant and marginal.[31]

American constructions of race and sexuality are conveyed repeatedly in the world of AIDS prevention and politics, teaching the racial and sexual rules of normalcy and marginality in America. These rules are part of the ideological backbone of racism. They reinforce the psychological and social processes that continue to obstruct the possibility of a democratic, tolerant, and peaceful life for all Americans. We can hope that if progressive straight and gay AIDS activists developed conscious awareness of these processes, how they operate, and their consequences, we might see a change toward not only graphic but also social inclusion and community.

When AIDS messages are beamed and distributed in the millions, they teach Americans about sexuality. This teaching is done as powerfully as the law and local customs will allow, because the teachers feel that they are teaching a life-and-death subject. If the students learn it right, they will live. If they don't, they will die. Consequently, much emotion goes into the planning and teaching. The images and stories and education are designed to be powerful. Yet more is being taught than sexual education or sexual change: sexual education is embedded in gender—and vice versa. It is also embedded in the social order in terms of other organizing principles: sexual education teaches about class, ethnicity, culture, language, racial conceptions, and family organization. Similarly, these social forms also teach us how we should be sexually. AIDS educators are teaching us American lessons about the racial aspects of our sexuality.

Clearly there is educational value in representing communities and not merely populations of people defined by sexually risky behavior. Ethnicity, culture, and community do reflect racial divisions. But the idealized vision of racial purity for Europeans and, by extension, for other of America's socially, constructed racial groupings is not accurate even within a racialized society, because boundaries are always blurred and violated. Very light- and very dark-skinned people of African descent are found in every African American neighborhood. Interracial families, couples, and encounters are also everywhere. Children with parents from two or more ethnic backgrounds are increasingly common. AIDS materials that occasionally depicted interracial heterosexuality, including interracial family life, would simply and appropriately reflect the reality of American society. The social and political construction of race and identity may reflect idealized views of the world. It can also be part of attempts to gain political or social power. But to be understood as applicable to their audiences, AIDS prevention images should reflect the social realities of life as well, and these realities include the sometimes taboo fact that interracial sex occurs in all neighborhoods and among all sexualities.

The Color of Money

City-wide competition for funding and programmatic control in San Francisco with regard to AIDS services for minority communities increased steadily between 1985 and 1988. The politicization of this competition culminated in intervention by the state Department of Health Services. For the first time funds that were previously given to the city Department of Public Health and then to SFAF to distribute to whomever it saw fit were granted directly to agencies in minority communities. The change in funding patterns was, oddly enough, the combined result of community-based activism and Republican hostility to the liberal policies of San Francisco's city government.

During the earlier years, the issue of the Foundation's relation to the minority communities in San Francisco was raised repeatedly. The May 1985 issue of the monthly newsletter of the Alice B. Toklas Lesbian and Gay Democratic Club contained a critical article by Norm Nickens, then chair of the AIDS and gay advisory committees of the city's Human Rights Commission. He reported:

> The best defense against AIDS is information, and this information is not reaching at-risk ethnic minority communities in San Francisco.
> Over the course of the last year, members of the Third World Caucus [of Alice] have met with representatives of the San Francisco AIDS Foundation to discuss the provision of AIDS information and educational services to at-risk ethnic minority communities. Despite these meetings, the Foundation has yet to come forth with an educational program designed to reach these communities. The Human Rights Commission recently voted to express its concern to the Health Commission over the failure of the Foundation to develop programs designed to outreach to ethnic minority communi-

ties, and called upon the Foundation to develop an affirmative action plan for the staff of the Foundation; the current staff of twenty-two has only two Third World people.

The next Alice meeting will feature a discussion of the impact of AIDS on ethnic minority communities, particularly Blacks and Latinos . . . . The Alice Third World Caucus will present recommendations designed to address the problem of outreach to ethnic minority communities in San Francisco and the problem of the representation of Third World people on the staff of the Foundation.[32]

When the forum was held, I spoke about risks to women.[33] Although I came from the Foundation, I do not remember being treated as an enemy, but rather as an ally who supported the concerns of the Caucus.

In April, I had heard Florence Stroud, the African American deputy director of the Department of Public Health (DPH) and the person responsible for community programs, discuss outreach to teenagers, with an emphasis on all teens and in particular reaching teenagers from ethnic minority backgrounds. Since we at the Women's Program had been discussing the importance of reaching both male and female youth about sexual risk, I told her we would send a proposal for a multi-ethnic outreach plan. The proposal mailed to her that May was based on a community organizing model, with each ethnic community the site of an organizing strategy. The steps were to include a meeting with community leaders, development of a task force that would make a strategic plan, and implementation of the plan.[34] Stroud responded that she had forwarded the proposal to Gary Titus in the AIDS Activity Office, which coordinated all AIDS education for the city, and to Dean Echenberg, the Bureau Chief for Disease Control. She added, "After we have had an opportunity to discuss your proposal more fully, I will get back to you."[35]

We never again heard from the DPH about the proposal. I was a white lesbian in a predominantly white male organization and, although I was the coordinator of the Women's AIDS Network and the director of the Women's Program at SFAF, our proposal was not submitted by a group representing any specific ethnic community. One could speculate that it was ignored for this reason. Still it was not the only such proposal to fall on deaf ears somewhere in the San Francisco's AIDS office.

From the first months that the epidemic surfaced in San Francisco, its impact had been felt among African Americans and, increasingly, in the Latino, Native American, Asian, and Pacific Islander populations. Nevertheless, the money for HIV prevention and care was managed almost exclusively by whites in white-controlled institutions. One contributing factor to this racial hegemony was the state's funding process.

The state had been following a rule that each political unit (city or county) would receive only one grant, typically through its health department, which would then parcel out the money to specific programs and agencies that would deliver services. From the state's point of view, the block-grant approach made management of the grant process easier. In San Francisco this meant that DPH

gave community money to the AIDS Foundation for prevention and social services and to Shanti for personal assistance and housing. Both agencies were run
by white, gay men.

Local minority community agencies and advocates in San Francisco became
increasingly angry because they wanted to provide their own services (education,
prevention, and care) instead of having to use these white gay organizations. The
primary issue was cultural sensitivity—or in 1990s jargon—"cultural competen-
cy." Many of the minority community HIV advocates were gay. Competition for
funds for heterosexuals within communities of color also became an issue. This
concern was ultimately mixed up with charges of homophobia from some members of the existing (white-dominated) AIDS agencies, which were staffed and
managed primarily by gay men and lesbians.

Added to an increasingly volatile situation were the composition and the policies of the AIDS Office of the San Francisco Department of Public Health. It and
all the department's allied departments (Sexually Transmitted Disease Control,
for example) were run by white men. In addition, the Health Commission, whose
job was to set policy for the department and to approve the health budget of the
city, included no people of color, despite the fact that San Francisco's population
was over 50 percent non-white.

As tensions escalated in 1986, a Minority Task Force on AIDS was formed by
Hank Tavera and other activists. It met with African Americans, Latinos, Asian
Americans, Native Americans, and women. Cheri Pies, the (white) coordinator of
AIDS education programs for the city at that time, tried to set up a meeting
between the community representatives and the head of the AIDS Office. When
the time came for the meeting and the community groups arrived, Jeff Amory,
director of the AIDS Office, did not show up, claiming later that he had not
thought the meeting was important. This angered the community groups so
much that they went straight to the state government. The state granting agency,
then under the control of a Republican governor, was happy to find an excuse to
reduce some of the power of the Democrat-controlled administration of San
Francisco.

In November 1986, the California Department of Health Services issued a
"Request for Proposals" for six pilot projects for "Underserved Minority
Populations." Three grants were to go to Los Angeles, and one each to San
Francisco, Alameda, and San Diego counties.[36] This was the first time that the
state had provided funds directly to agencies within a county and not to a local
health department for distribution. This move was intended to circumvent local
health department priorities and policy making. In addition, it provided several
important political gains to the state government: The state Department of
Health Services was able to align itself with minorities challenging white (and
gay) leadership, and it was able to take a swipe at the more progressive governments of the counties where it would send money (up to $100,000 per project)
by sending dollars to a specific agency within the supposedly coordinated area

under the local health department or its lead agencies.

The state granted funds to three San Francisco minority agencies: the Black Coalition on AIDS, the Minority AIDS Task Force, and the California Prostitutes Education Project. From that moment on, public prevention funds for minority communities in San Francisco went to agencies directly representing the communities; the AIDS Foundation's hegemony was broken. Within a year, several more agencies focused on AIDS issues in the Latino, Native American, and Asian American communities came into being and were also receiving funds from the state.

After the re-allocation of state funds directly to the minority organizations, the channeling and control of state prevention monies through SFAF for minority outreach was over. Nevertheless the agency continued to be one of the city's most important AIDS agencies. Its board raised ever-larger proportions of its budget from non-government sources and the Foundation became an ally of the minority organizations by transfering skills and advocating for the poor and for immigrants, two groups of special concern to the minority organizations.

As the first HIV prevention organization in its city, the San Francisco AIDS Foundation had the opportunity not only to grow rapidly from the start, but also to establish relative hegemony over the field of HIV education, prevention, and services in the city. Its leaders seized upon this opportunity, initially sharing portions of the public funding pie with Shanti (direct care and housing for those who were ill) and the AIDS Health Project (mental health services).

The Foundation's decision to provide services and education to "everyone" meant that it could create new departments or "bureaus" as new funds and areas of intervention were discovered. This set the stage for its broad claims of expertise and continuing expansion. It also provided a rationale for the development of a variety of programs for population subgroups (heterosexuals, people of color, "the general population") that were not extensively represented on the staff, administration, or board of the organization.

This approach and the resulting bureaucratic expansion had consequences for the Foundation. For one thing, it became more moderate within the overall spectrum of AIDS activism. Because its leaders often interacted with state and federal policy makers and wanted to be viewed as "experts," they toned down their rhetoric and occasionally found themselves supporting more moderate positions than their staff would have liked. The Foundation was able, however, to keep some of its radical edge by increasingly raising its own funds and relying less and less on public funding. During the nineties, it has consistently raised over half its budget from non-governmental sources. This enabled it to continue to play an active role in public policy.

Also, its broad reach made the organization susceptible to charges of working in areas where it was not knowledgeable. Thus, it faced competition and criticism for providing materials and services to people of color, various language groups, teenagers, drug users, heterosexuals, even gay men. These charges were expressed as accusations of racism and sexism, although it might be more accurate to say that the Foundation simply was not as sophisticated in every area of specialization as groups representing these populations could be. Lastly, the Foundation's desire (or need—for fundraising purposes) to be part of the local elite may have caused it to tone down its message. In all these areas, the Foundation adopted what I would call a white, male, and gay standpoint, albeit liberal.

While the San Francisco AIDS Foundation lost its status as a "radical" organization because of its growth and bureaucratization, it increased in power and influence, which it used to protect people with HIV and to advocate for them. The Foundation was effective precisely because of its size, strength and legitimacy. On the other hand, to achieve these goals it had to betray the vision of consensus and the prioritization of experience over professionalism shared by those who founded it. In this, SFAF is not alone. As we shall see, parallel conflicts between theory and practice also occurred in Cal-PEP and Prevention Point. Meanwhile, in that same year of 1987 in San Francisco, gay Asian Americans were struggling for the same visibility and AIDS funding that white men had secured five years earlier.

Becoming Visible:
Asian Americans

The development of Asian-American responses to the HIV/AIDS epidemic has been a struggle for visibility and particularity within an epidemic in which Asians and Pacific Islanders were first invisible and then seen as monocultural by dominant institutions. This chapter provides a short history of the early AIDS epidemic in the San Francisco Bay area as it affected Asian and Pacific Islander communities.[1] This history was one of multiple struggles for visibility: first, to be acknowledged by researchers and funders as communities with real risks for HIV and, second, against monocultural stereotypes. Through this process, gay men in these communities and those with HIV have ceased to be bystanders and have become leaders.

The Asian AIDS Task Force invented itself in 1986. It was made up of service providers, individual members, and volunteers who got together to find out what types of services Asians needed, to advocate for funds, and to produce a needs assessment.[2] There were no Asian/Pacific prevention activities at this time. The Task Force became the Asian/Pacific AIDS Coalition (A/PAC); its purpose was advocacy, lobbying for funds, cooperation, and formative research regarding the Asian and Pacific Islander communities. One educator commented that, in 1986,

> there was a huge discrepancy in how AIDS dollars were allocated to our Asian communities to do education, as compared to who was infected by the epidemic, who was coming down with HIV. Most of the dollars going to prevention/education [were] being spent on doing general community education. Nice brochures that didn't talk about homosexuality at all, or if they did it was a certain type of reference, and people were using the money to go to classes just to talk about AIDS without really targeting information to gay/bisexual men. It was truly a limitation with the resources that we had. The bigger question for us was, Why don't you have gay and bisexual men working in your agency so that you could do that type of work?[2a]

In 1987, the Asian AIDS Project was the first organization to get a small amount of funding to provide AIDS services for Asian Americans. The Project hired several health educators who were either openly gay or still in the closet. All those on the board of the directors, ironically, were straight men. Their ability to imagine appropriate interventions was limited by their lack of gay experience. The directors also had to overcome the barriers of homophobia.[3]

The Gay Asian Pacific Alliance (GAPA) joined the Coalition in 1987; soon GAPA decided that it would be more effective in providing services through its own organization. In 1989, the GAPA-Community HIV Project (G-CHP) emerged from GAPA with a goal of developing a more activist-based program and incorporating more gay men in administration. Although they had not yet received specific funding, they organized workshops. Steve Lew participated in these early efforts:

> I was probably one of the earlier persons that was public about my HIV status . . . . Just by doing a few things we created a nucleus in our community for gay/bisexual men.[4]

The second year, G-CHP got funding for prevention services, which helped them to establish an agency. Volunteers were recruited and a buddy program started. Vince Sales reflects on his awareness of AIDS as a former AIDS volunteer:

> I met the first HIV-positive Asian/Pacific Islander and I was completely blown away by it. It was such a powerful experience, I couldn't sleep. I had to talk to someone about it because it just overwhelmed me. It's such a fearsome kind of disease, and there were misconceptions surrounding it. I wanted to take hold of that fear by educating myself.

That same year, Jim Naritomi started an AIDS education program within the Japanese Community Youth Council (JCYC) with $24,000, which was spent on salaries, operational expenses, and the development and production of Japanese bilingual AIDS brochures.

> At the time, my other half (I'm gay) had AIDS. I was kind of a bit down all the time. We had a kid. The executive director of the Japanese Community Youth Council, who was also a friend and relative, came to me, and we talked many times about starting this Japanese program. AIDS/HIV is too close to me. With Jerry dying, I lost many friends, probably will lose more.
>
> When Jerry was still alive we talked about it. He said to do it temporarily. It was supposed to be only a six-month arrangement, and I'm still here. I think a part of it was that I was extremely frustrated within the first six months because I worked extremely hard. It was very difficult to develop everything from scratch. People weren't ready to talk about HIV. This was 1987. Individually they supported me for the person I am. There's a difference between personal support versus proactive support. It took some time before the proactive support came, but it did take its toll in its very beginning. And I'm still here.

Steve Lew was open and honest about his decision to take part in AIDS education. With a sigh he commented:

> For the most part it feels very empowering, because a lot of the reason I got involved in activism around HIV is because I knew I was positive. I tested back in 1986. A lot of the feelings that I went through were feelings of powerlessness, feelings that I had no

control of the situation. At the time that I tested there was very little information known about how you could treat HIV. That's still the case now; they still don't know what's really effective. But they have options; there's some treatment. But at that time there were so many unknowns and even in terms of knowing how long people could live a healthy life.

That's changed a bit now because I've lived a healthy life since then, and I still feel like I have much more of a long-term vision for myself. So I can focus on HIV education not only in terms of prevention, but also working with people who are sick, helping them to see how they can cope with a life-threatening disease. Sometimes it gets a little difficult because it's hard not to separate out talking and living with the disease and at some point feeling that it saturates your whole life. And sometimes seeing other people get sick does push the button too, because then I think, Well is this going to happen to me? And you go through a whole personalization of it, too. But for the most part I feel that it's been a very good decision for me and that it's really helped me to confront a lot of my own issues.

In 1990, the Asian American Communities Against AIDS (AACAA) was initiated by Naritomi to campaign for a larger pot of money. The money was then divided evenly among the five consortium members to start HIV programs: Chinese AIDS Prevention Project, Japanese Against AIDS Project, West Bay Filipino AIDS Project, Southeast Asian AIDS Prevention Project, and at the Korean Community Service Center. Naritomi commented:

The problem is because we're one project [AACAA] we don't like to give the idea that we all do the same things the same way equally and identically. The communities that are involved have different expertise. Additionally, the people who work in prevention programs within different communities have different barriers, different successes. They're not all the same.

Naritomi went on to say that the Filipino and Japanese communities were currently the most progressive of his consortium members due to their consistent staffing and the linkages that they have formed in the community.

Culture and Risk

When Christine Wong contacted the Korean Community Service Center in 1993, she was surprised to find that there were only a few pamphlets available in Korean. When a worker at the Center was asked why no program had been initiated, he replied that there had been no interest in the Korean community to start one. We asked staff at other organizations why they thought that the Korean Community Service Center had not started an AIDS program. One person suggested that Koreans did not want to be active in the consortium, even though the Center is a member of AACAA. This AIDS educator mused that Koreans in San Francisco might feel that there are not enough people infected in order to make it worthwhile to seek funds.

Nevertheless, most other Asian community-based organizations in San Francisco had begun to develop culturally relevant HIV/AIDS material by 1993. Initially, these HIV education programs were located in already-existing (straight) Asian non-profit agencies. When funding was first available, in the late 1980s, the agencies chose or were pressured by Asian gay activists to incorporate HIV/AIDS education programs into their services. Gradually the programs, their locations, and the demographic characteristics of the providers have shifted. The brochures and pamphlets, the workshops, and the educators have changed along with the epidemic to become more of a reflection of their targeted communities. As suggested by Robert Bernardo from the Asian AIDS Project's "Love Like This" Theater Project, "The more friends see people on stage that are like them, the more they are willing to listen to them." Fatima Angeles agreed and commented, "We want to target young Filipino kids. My educators are young and Filipino. So automatically there's a connection, automatically there's a bond."

In 1993, the three most important service and prevention organizations for Asian/Pacific Islanders in the San Francisco Bay area were GAPA Community HIV Project, Asian AIDS Project, and the Filipino Task Force on AIDS, all run by gay and bisexual men. Although many of the suburbs of San Francisco have large Asian populations there are few prevention programs for their Asian and Pacific Islander communities. This may be due to a number of factors: the relatively low number of AIDS cases among Asians and Pacific Islanders, a lack of knowledge of services or funding sources, a lack of culturally appropriate services (i.e., bilingual, bicultural, sensitive to Asians and Pacific Islanders), and the limited funding available to support such ongoing education and programs. "You must have an enormous [AIDS] funding base in order to have a staff that is bicultural, bilingual, and biliterate," Naritomi noted. Even in San Francisco where there is a long history of community-based HIV organizations, ethnic minorities continue to struggle with barriers of racism, lack of economic power, homophobia, and sexism. According to Sales, "When it [the Asian AIDS Project] started, everyone wanted to see AAP fall flat on its face. It had a reputation of being homophobic. If you want to serve people at risk for HIV, you can't be judgmental."[5]

The few community-based organizations in San Francisco that were doing outreach to Asians and Pacific Islanders were centered around gay and bisexual Asian men. However, there was little outreach to lesbian, bisexual, or straight women or to transgender or transvestite Asians and Pacific Islanders. While there were campaigns that did target other populations besides gay or bisexual men, their programs were not as rigorous nor readily available. This may represent the slow growth of awareness in the broader Asian community.

The Asian community's response to AIDS has been seriously delayed by a number of myths, all to the effect that, as one epidemiologist put it as early as 1983, Asians are "immune" to AIDS.[6] It is more likely that Asians have been infected with HIV since the first cases were diagnosed in the United States in 1981, but that a low level of incidence produced misunderstandings and late and missed diagnoses. Nevertheless, many Asians believed these early articles that denied the existence of AIDS among Asian Americans. Therefore they did not perceive themselves as susceptible.

The lack of accurate information on AIDS incidence may have reinforced misconceptions that Asians hold about HIV. Even by 1996 few articles had been published that specifically addressed the issue of Asians and AIDS in the U.S.; even fewer had been written on Asians with AIDS. In addition, AIDS intersects with several taboo topics in Asian culture—sex, illness, death, and homosexuality. This intersection poses a further educational barrier.

In the 1980s, most of the AIDS education materials available to Asians were translations of materials originally designed for populations with a high level of English literacy. Pictures and diagrams of AIDS epidemiology and illness progression were very complex. If there were drawings or photos, the people did not look Asian.

It is likely that many Asian Americans ignored or did not take the materials seriously. To make matters worse, health educators were primarily white men who did not speak the languages with which Asians were familiar. This made it even harder for Asian Americans to understand what these dominant figures were trying to tell them. As a result, AIDS education among Asians in the first five years of the epidemic was relatively unsuccessful.

Of all the stereotypes concerning Asians, the "model minority" myth has probably been most damaging in terms of AIDS awareness. This stereotype, which has repeatedly been presented in mainstream media, portrays the Asian American as successful, compliant, quiet, and subservient. Other ethnic groups have often compared themselves to the Asian and Pacific Islander community by saying, "Why can't we be like them?" thus setting up Asians as fit targets for resentment. Asians and Pacific Islanders are seen as "foreigners" and a threat, rather than an addition to American society. Vi Huynh of the Chinatown Youth Center suggests that "society drives them (youth) into losing their identity, and they, therefore, remove themselves from Asian culture . . . . Parents may have a rude awakening."[7] This myth may also create additional pressure on youth from their families to "do good."

The model-minority myth about Asians includes the belief that they do not engage in promiscuous sex, drugs, or illegal acts. But these activities do exist. Some of the more serious problems in the Asian and Pacific Islander communities include poverty, substance abuse, mental illness, and domestic violence.[8] The Tenderloin area of San Francisco, where many first-generation Asians reside, is also home to a concentration of brothels and on-street prostitution. As Jim Naritomi commented:

> We should acknowledge that Asians, as a whole, have achieved a great deal of financial success as a result of educational pursuits and business endeavors . . . . The bottom line is, that's all wonderful. Sounds like painting a rosy picture and it is. We shouldn't deny that part. But we also have a large population of people, whether they be immigrants or U.S. born, who don't have an educational advantage or who may not have had any

formal educational at all. Immigrants and refugees never finished high school, as we know. They don't say that though. We have this image to continue.[9]

The belief that AIDS is a "white, gay" disease and not a pandemic problem has two important effects within Asian American communities. It limits effective services to Asian Americans who are HIV-positive, and it leads to the further spread of HIV.

Kevin Fong, director of the Asian Health Services' AIDS Project in Oakland, noted that parents are unwilling to admit that their children are having sex. But in order to prevent HIV infection in teens, Ginny Bourassa, coordinator of youth programs for even the same organization, had to acknowledge the opposite: Teens were having sex. She integrated education, self-esteem, negotiation skills, and responsibility into her training of HIV/AIDS peer educators. She argued that "young women are getting pregnant, and they have to assume responsibility . . . . We need to get education out to men, too . . . . They need to get communication going." If you can get pregnant, she explains, you must be having sex, and you can get AIDS, since sperm and HIV are transmitted the same way.

Homosexuality is disapproved of both publicly and within families. It is looked down upon especially because it prevents marriage and procreation in a culture where a man's primary obligation is to carry on the family name through marriage and children. Homosexuality also represents deviant and disapproved sexual behavior. This combination of disapproval and stigmatization may lead many gay, lesbian, and bisexual Asian Americans to hide their sexual identities.

According to Bart Aoki, of Asian American Recovery Services, another challenge arises when trying to educate Asian substance abusers. The difficulty lies in finding out who the substance abusers are, where they are located, and which substances they use. Aoki claimed that he did not make the assumption that all Asians and Pacific Islanders "users" shoot up because "that would be wrong and only help to encourage Asians to try other methods of using drugs." Of the Asian drug users in San Francisco coming to its program, the Asian American Recovery Service has found that there are more Filipino and Japanese than Chinese intravenous drug users. At the time of our study, no research had been done on whether Asian drug users use only their own needles when shooting up. However, one can assume that at least some shoot up and share needles with other Asians or members of other ethnic groups. Socially dominant users usually use the needle first, followed by the other, less dominant users which, according to Aoki, include Asians and Pacific Islanders.[10] "They are out there; they're just harder to find," Aoki stressed.

Another impediment to effective AIDS organizing in Asian American communities is a tendency to aggregate the very heterogeneous communities that make up the U.S. Asian and Pacific Islander populations. Categorizing different Asian ethnic groups into one homogeneous group overlooks the fact that there are diverse languages, cultures, beliefs, and traditions within each national and ethnic category, as well as historic diversity. According to the 1990 U.S. Census

Bureau, there are 210,876 (29.1 percent of the population) Asians and Pacific Islanders in San Francisco City and County.[11] Eighteen distinct groups were identified in the census. At least thirty-two different Asian languages and dialects are spoken in the Bay Area. There is also great variety in religious beliefs, number of generations in the United States, sexuality, roles within the family structure, gender issues, socioeconomic class, and generational differences.[12]

Despite these differences, there are some strong similarities among Asian American cultures. One's family and community play a major role in one's life in such a way that they frequently override the individual's needs. A person is seen more as a representative of his or her family and less as an individual.[13] One must protect "face," for its loss will be reflected upon the individual's family and community.

It has been more than a decade since the epidemiologist speaking at one of the first public AIDS conferences in San Francisco stated that Asians were immune to AIDS.[14] At that time, in 1983, there were no reported cases among Asians. Even today, the number is still relatively small, indicating that the epidemic among Asians and Pacific Islanders in the U.S. is in its early stages. The epidemic is mushrooming throughout Asia, however.[15]

Although Asians and Pacific Islanders comprise about 30 percent of San Francisco's population, they contributed only 2.4 percent of the cumulative AIDS caseload by 1995. According to John Newmeyer, writing in *Mid-City Numbers*, a monthly bulletin of AIDS statistics, "Unless A/PI AIDS cases are badly unreported—which I consider very unlikely—we must conclude that the disease has affected A/PIs in our part of the world far less than it has affected the other major ethnic groups."[16]

The city's Asian and Pacific Islander cumulative AIDS caseload is 9 percent female, much higher than for whites or Latinos, but much lower than for blacks. Most of the Asian and Pacific Islander AIDS caseload (80 percent) appear to have male-to-male sex as the sole risk factor. An additional 80 percent reported injection drug use as a risk factor; half of these were men who had sex with men. Notably, the intravenous drug user risk factor is rarer in the Asian and Pacific Islander caseload than in that of blacks (38 percent), Latinos (15 percent), or whites (12 percent). However, Asians and Pacific Islanders were only 40 out of 3,191 (1.3 percent) San Francisco AIDS cases with intravenous drug user histories. Newmeyer examined the possibility that these figures—for HIV diagnoses and for intravenous drug user risk—might be wrong, perhaps because Asians were reluctant to seek help. To test these theories he reviewed emergency room and coroner reports and concluded that the drugs most frequently used are less likely to be injectable and that the HIV infection rates are fairly accurate.

Until 1988, Asian and Pacific Islander AIDS cases were categorized into a group labeled "other." Since then, they have been identified as a distinct race/ethnic group. Further breakdowns by culture indicate that Filipinos have the highest rates of infection among Asian/Pacific Islanders in San Francisco.[17] Nationally, among Filipinos, the highest incidence rate is in San Francisco, followed by Los Angeles, and then Hawaii. In San Francisco, Chinese incidence rates are some-what less than those for Filipinos, followed in turn by Japanese.[18]

In his 1995 analysis, Newmeyer also compared rates of HIV disease among Asian Americans and Pacific Islanders. He noted that two-thirds of the Asian and Pacific Islander caseload had been reported among two ethnic communities, Filipinos and Chinese. Here is his table comparing intra-Asian and Pacific Islander AIDS cases, to the city's Asian and Pacific Islander population as a whole:[18a]

	A/PI AIDS Caseload	City A/PI Population
Filipino	39.0%	19.0%
Chinese	27.0%	62.0%
Japanese	13.0%	5.5%
Pacific Islander	7.0%	1.5%
Southeast Asian	6.0%	5.5%
Korean	1.0%	3.0%
Other	6.0%	3.5%

Source: John Newmeyer, *Mid-City Numbers,* Vol. 8 (April 1995).

AIDS had thus affected Filipinos, Japanese, and Pacific Islanders relatively more, and Chinese and Koreans relatively less.

HIV serosurveillance also showed low rates of infection among Asians and Pacific Islanders in San Francisco. Asian and Pacific Islander HIV+ rates were 3.1 percent at sexually transmitted disease clinics, 2.0 percent at methadone pro-grams, 2.2 percent at outpatient detox programs, and zero percent among mili-tary recruits. In all four of these populations, Asian and Pacific Islander HIV+ rates were significantly less than those for whites, blacks, or Latinos.

For California as a whole, Asians and Pacific Islanders are just as underrepre-sented in HIV infection rates as in San Francisco, compared to other ethnic groups. Here are data from Newmeyer's study on Californians living with AIDS as of mid-1994, shown by rates per 100,000 residents of the particular gender and ethnicity:

	Males	Females
Blacks	386	62
Whites	184	8
Latinos	119	11
A/PIs	47	5

Source: John Newmeyer, *Mid-City Numbers,* Vol. 8 (April 1995).

Steve Lew, director of education programs of the Gay Asian Pacific Alliance Community HIV Project, commented on these trends in 1993: "The Japanese community is not that big and yet the cases show they're the third largest group of people [infected]. Their incidence is very high. We don't know why . . . . Overall it's hard to draw a definite conclusion in terms of ethnicity." Although Asian and Pacific Islander rates of AIDS vary among cities and states, little research has been done to understand the patterns.

One approach to understanding these patterns of infection is to collect data on rates of HIV testing. HIV anonymous test sites provide a complementary data source to AIDS diagnoses for assessing the spread of the epidemic among Asian Americans and Pacific Islanders. Vi Huynh, case manager of the Chinatown Youth Center, is also a pre- and post-HIV test counselor at Health Center One in San Francisco. He reported feeling like a "gatekeeper" because he was responsible for revealing to his patients that their fate was in the hands of AIDS. Huynh estimated that of the clients he counseled in San Francisco, only about 10 percent of the Asians who came to the center were there to be tested. He was alarmed that out of the forty confidential and anonymous test sites available in San Francisco, there were few Asians going in for HIV testing, especially since the sites are near locations where many immigrants reside. Lew suggested one possible reason might be that Asians do not trust government agencies. Many believe the forms filled out prior to testing—even at anonymous test sites—may later be used as evidence against them.

If Asian Americans are less likely to go in for testing or care even after an AIDS diagnosis and symptoms have appeared, the epidemic will be more hidden. Many Asians and Pacific Islanders diagnosed with HIV wait until their illness is well-advanced before initiating a first encounter with a health care provider, usually in the emergency room.[19] Because a family member's illness is a reflection on all, a family will often try to hide the patient in his or her last stages of AIDS in order to avoid being stigmatized by the extended family, friends, or the broader community. Death certificates may then state the cause of death as cancer or pneumonia. With such diagnoses, the deaths are not reported to the Centers for Disease Control,[20] which leads to further undercounting. Naritomi commented,

> They don't go in until they have symptoms. Very few come in for help until they are very sick. They've already exhausted all of their resources. By resources, I mean they've allowed, if they have insurance, their insurance to cancel because they can't afford it. They've gone hungry. Many have not sought medical care or charged it to their insurance and therefore have depleted their financing because they don't want their insurance company or their employer to know their HIV status.[21]

The highest number of sexually transmitted disease cases reported among foreign students is among Japanese students, according to Ippei Yasuda, health educator at the Japanese Against AIDS Project. He added that Japanese foreign students seek abortion the most, which indicates these women are not using condoms or other barrier methods that prevent both conception and HIV transmission. Yasuda hypothesized that the apparently high level of sexual activity without barrier protection may stem from strong family restrictions in Japan, followed by a sense of freedom on arrival in the U.S., allowing both male and female students to try activities that were restricted before.[22]

Newly arrived immigrants have been shown to be the least knowledgeable Asians on the subject of AIDS. The articles in Asian newspapers often downplay AIDS and rarely discuss prevention methods. Even when HIV/AIDS materials are translated into an Asian language, it is the language of only one community. Many Asian immigrants tend to trust broadcast media and some believe that if a reporter is on television her comments must have been approved and so must be correct. In addition, lack of understanding of the U.S. health care system, social service benefits, and lack of insurance leave many immigrants without access to health care and health education. Vince Sales explained that,

> Some [immigrants] have fatalistic attitudes toward HIV. I think it underlies the whole attitude of Asians toward prevention. When we seek medical care, it's more for treatment. We're not there to prevent it. It's more like, "cure me," and we look at medical doctors as experts to cure whatever we have. We don't necessarily think of medicine as prevention. Medicine in the Third World is expensive. We don't think in those terms.

According to Sales, "many immigrants believe that HIV is an airborne disease . . . since this is how many well-known diseases are spread in Third World countries."[23] Naritomi added, "You're always going to have people that are going to resist [understanding HIV transmission]. That's going to be forevermore. It's not going to be absolute." Yasuda commented that there is a popular Japanese saying that goes, "Something which stinks, put the lid on it!"

The KABB Studies

With this much active avoidance within the Asian/Pacific communities, it was inevitable that the progress of the epidemic would be seriously misunderstood and understated. Thus, when public funding for services to ethnic and racial minority communities became available in the late 1980s, Asian/Pacific AIDS activists were seriously disadvantaged in making their case for a need within their communities.

In order to receive funding from public sources, community agencies must demonstrate need. The agencies usually begin with a needs assessment, as the San Francisco AIDS Foundation did when beginning its women's services. To get funds for their communities, Asian and Pacific Islander activists had to follow the same route.

During the late 1980s and early 1990s, many studies of racial and ethnic minority communities were conducted in order to qualify for public health funding. Typically they consisted of telephone interviews or door-to-door surveys concerning knowledge, attitudes, behaviors, and beliefs (KABB). Several of the Asian American and Pacific Islander AIDS agencies currently operating in San Francisco were funded as a result of studies conducted in 1989-1990. These studies are important for several reasons. First, they are part of the tangible results of the ethnic AIDS revolt of 1987, fulfilling part of the minority community demand for research. Second, they represent the public shape of Asian and Pacific Islander HIV risk both to their own communities and to public health authorities and private foundations. Third, much current outreach is based on the findings in these studies. And fourth, unfortunately, they tell little about the social relations of sex and behavior change.

Despite, or perhaps, because of their use of standard survey techniques, some of the study results do not accurately correlate with other known facts about the populations surveyed. For example, the Filipino Knowledge, Attitudes, Behavior, and Beliefs (KABB) study found no Filipino intravenous drug users in San Francisco, which we know is incorrect. Therefore, from a scientific point of view, one must describe the San Francisco Asian and Pacific Islander studies (like many other such studies) as only suggestive, despite their quantitative style and scientific feel. From a sociological viewpoint, they are part of the process of becoming visible and gaining the power of legitimate representation.

One of the most important results of these studies of HIV/AIDS in Asian and Pacific Islander communities was to shed light on the many differences among them. Studies were conducted in the Filipino, Chinese, Japanese, and Southeast Asian communities.

Among Filipinos, overall knowledge about HIV transmission was poor. More than 40 percent of the sample held incorrect beliefs, such as that AIDS is caused by sharing toothbrushes or razors, by needles used for vaccinations or laboratory tests, by receiving blood transfusions after 1985, by donating blood, and via mosquito bites. Moreover, accurate knowledge about AIDS transmission did not correlate with reported changes in sexual behavior or the practice of risk reduction.[24]

Rene Astudillo, interim executive director of the Filipino Task Force on AIDS, estimated that about 80 percent of the total population of openly gay and bisexual Asian and Pacific Islander men are Filipino. There is a sense of freedom experienced by gay and bisexual immigrants when they arrive in the U.S., and they may engage in activities that they would not previously take part in. They often bring with them attitudes of denial, *hiya* (shame), and *bahala na* (come-what-may) which are part of Filipino culture.[25]

In the Chinese community there was a relatively high awareness of the existence of AIDS, but over half of the people interviewed reported that they knew little or nothing about it substantively. Nevertheless, 74 percent felt they could protect themselves from AIDS and that it probably would not affect their lives. And nearly everyone correctly identified all known ways of AIDS transmission, despite their claim to know little or nothing about the disease. Over half of the respondents felt people with AIDS should be quarantined, however, and 74 percent also felt that these people should not be identified publicly.[26]

Huynh stressed that, although regional differences were not explored in the KABB study, there are different attitudes about sex among Chinese Americans, depending on the area of Asia from which they emigrated. Those from mainland China are more shy, reserved, and not exposed as much to sex education. For them, according to Huynh, "Condoms mean sex and sex is taboo. Therefore, it shouldn't be discussed."[27] Immigrants from Hong Kong, on the other hand, are more assertive, current on AIDS, and will challenge the educator. Huynh added that those from mainland China found HIV more difficult to accept in their community, and he himself found it harder to talk to them about HIV transmission. He claimed that he had to talk "babyish." Many different names were substituted for various sexual activities because there were no Chinese language equivalents.

The results of the KABB study of the San Francisco Japanese community conducted in 1989 reveal subtle but important differences from other Asian populations. Ninety-five percent of the people interviewed had heard of AIDS, and almost half knew someone with AIDS. They identified all the known ways of HIV transmission (sexual contact, sharing needles, blood transfusion, and breast milk). However some were confused about casual transmission, believing that mosquito bites or drinking out of the same glass could infect a person. Like the Chinese, however, they felt able to protect themselves.[28]

According to Yasuda, in Japan, it is customary for the parents, usually the mother, to handle the sex education of the children.[29] However, youth in Japan and in the U.S. currently have more knowledge about sexuality than their parents. They learn mostly from other peers or through books. Yasuda complained that these books are sometimes factually wrong; also, some do not mention contraception. The different information levels can create barriers between parents and children. The child seeks to learn more from peers when parents do not want to discuss sex.

The Southeast Asian communities studied consisted of Cambodians, Laotians, and Vietnamese.[30] Here, too, a variety of incorrect beliefs was found, including that AIDS can be transmitted by kissing, sitting on toilet seats, and through insect bites. All three ethnic groups ranked AIDS as the second greatest health problem in the community; yet there was a sense that the threat of AIDS was not personal but was something that affects "other people."

Kyle Monroe-Spencer, a health educator from the Southeast Asian AIDS Project, commented that, "if Southeast Asians have concerns, they would rather go to mainstream AIDS organizations for fear that their information would not be kept confidential." This posed a problem because many of the mainstream

AIDS organizations, like the San Francisco AIDS Foundation, did not have bicultural educators or other staff who could speak the various ethnic Asian languages. Moreover, according to Monroe-Spencer, mainstream materials and services were not designed to be culturally sensitive to the needs of the Asian population. In contrast, she stated, the center for Southeast Asian Refugee Resettlement provided useful services, but these are not associated with HIV/AIDS in the minds of local residents.[31]

Monroe-Spencer continued: "Men mostly decide if they are going to use condoms, and women don't talk to men about it . . . . They [Vietnamese] didn't even know that they could go into a drug store and buy condoms." In comparing her project's experiences with the various Southeast Asian groups, Monroe-Spencer noted that HIV education in the ethnic Vietnamese community seemed to be more successful; she attributed this to more extensive experience with the population on the part of the educators. (Vietnamese are the largest of the Southeast Asian population groups in the San Francisco Bay Area.) There is much less access to subgroups of Vietnamese, according to Monroe-Spencer. She noted that Laotians had a more visible transgender population than did other Asian communities, and that gay and bisexual men among Southeast Asians were more open than their counterparts in other Asian countries.

As a result of the KABB studies and other findings, it was possible for activists to channel funding directly to community-based organizations in a way that was culturally sensitive for the first time. Asian/Pacific AIDS educators who worked with gay men were able to refine their approaches to accommodate subtle but important distinctions. For instance, as David Cho, community health specialist from the Asian Health Services' AIDS Project commented, not all gay or bisexual Asians identify themselves as such. These men would rather classify themselves as men who sometimes have sex with other men. Unfortunately, this may have put them at a higher risk because using condoms identified them as "gay" rather than as casual participants in male-to-male sex. New strategies were needed to deal with this identity issue.

Another risk in the Asian community, according to Yasuda, is that gay Japanese foreign students are more likely to be sexually passive because they lack English and consequently have ineffective negotiation skills.[32] They become the receptive partners, engaging in anal sex without a condom. He believed this passive behavior is especially characteristic of interracial relationships, and this generates an important risk of HIV infection for these students because their white partners already have high infection rates.[33] Although homosexuality is not typically accepted openly within a Japanese family, it is tolerated.[34] And, as with other sexual options, it is sometimes explored by visiting Japanese while in the United States.

Lew felt that many closeted gay Asians were not comfortable meeting people in openly gay environments.[35] Instead they went to places like public bathrooms, adult movie theaters, or adult book stores. They feel that these environments are more anonymous and therefore more private. However, Lew said, "These places are risky because people go there specifically for sex. So a lot of people will break down to just have sex. There is a lot of compromising without using condoms."[36]

According to Fatima Angeles, project coordinator of the Filipino AIDS Education Project,

> A lot of teenagers rely, not on their moms and dads, but they rely on their friends. It's just happened too many times that their friends had the wrong answers . . . . It's confusing for immigrant kids. It's doubly hard for kids who come from another country and have to come here and adjust. There's culture shock. There's also a language problem. Things are more open here. They get confused. They want to do what their parents want them to do, but they want to be accepted by their peers.[37]

In a study conducted by the Filipino Task Force in Vallejo (a Bay Area suburb) in 1993, it was found that one in four Filipino American teens had tried illegal drugs and three in four had drunk alcohol. Of those who admitted that they engage in sexual intercourse, almost half responded that they did not use a condom the last time they had sex, although virtually all of them knew that unprotected sex can transmit the HIV virus.[38] Most of those interviewed were between fifteen and seventeen years old. Of the teens she works with, Angeles commented,

> . . . They want to play the numbers game, because they want to feel good. They ask questions like, "What are the chances of me playing basketball and I get infected if blood gets into my eye?" They don't think they're at risk. It's really important that Magic Johnson came out because he wasn't white and had HIV. For that man to have gotten HIV from unprotected sex, that just proves it's not safe. They're young. They haven't dealt with death and dying. They have other things to look forward to. It's not in their heads.

First- and second-generation youth are seen as especially in need of attention. Huynh commented that Asian young people "don't have a culture of their own . . . their own identity."[39] Several educators commented that the sub-population that engages in the most risky behaviors and needs most direct attention are young gay men. As Lew put it,

> This is a city [San Francisco] where a lot of young gay and bisexual men liberate to. It's a very expensive city to live in and yet there's this closer feeling that it's a supportive place for gay people, that a lot of them end up really needing to have sex for survival purposes . . . doing sex for money or to find a roommate.[40]

Prevention Strategies

HIV/AIDS education to Asians and Pacific Islanders had just begun. The Gay Asian Pacific Alliance Community HIV Project designed a postcard-style booklet to deal with issues of anonymity, safe sex, and cruising. It was called "Safer Sex Comes in All Languages" and focused on ways that gay and bisexual men could talk to their partners about safer sex. G-CHP asked people to write stories in Chinese, Japanese, Thai, Pidgin, Filipino, Cambodian, Korean, and Vietnamese; all were translated into English as well. One of the postcard stories took place in a public restroom where people occasionally meet to have sex. The main character, Japanese, tells about "cruising" someone who wouldn't use a condom so he left. He did what was right, he says. He'll just wait for the next person to come along.

According to Lew, "G-CHP tries to pick up a lot of situations that we know happen. We're not necessarily saying that this is the way we always want people to do things, but we realize that this is the reality for how a lot of gay men are sexually active. We want them to know those skills in whatever context."

G-CHP also held gay social events that included, for instance, condom corsages or a tunnel of love in which there were interactive games that taught negotiation skills. Lew says, "A lot of people in our community only relate to each other in the bars socially, so the best place to sort of create an atmosphere for HIV education is linking it to their own lives by doing social events."

The number of community-based programs was still not adequate. Though there were some educational programs for Asian and Pacific Islander heterosexuals and youth, programs specifically for women, people with disabilities, children, substance abusers, and sex industry workers were yet to be developed.[41] The diversity that is common to any ethnic minority community poses difficult challenges. AIDS education for Asians has changed over the years to become more "culturally sensitive," but, as Steve Lew commented on the notion of cultural sensitivity, "The whole idea of culturally appropriate, culturally competent and culturally specific is that it usually referred to the context of people of color." Organizations such as G-CHP, Lew says, are drawing much finer distinctions, to

> "broaden the definition to include anything that creates a cultural identification as well as a way to include sub-groups of culture, i.e., in order to be culturally competent you need to address gays, lesbians or bisexuals, possibly people who are disabled, and different sections within a community. We really try to use resources to address cultural competency from looking at people who we are working with, try to develop different cultural aspects that are important to them."

The services that were provided did not even meet the linguistic needs of the Asian and Pacific Islander community. For example, Ippei Yasuda from the Japanese American AIDS Project was the only member of the staff who spoke Japanese and therefore acted not only as an educator but as a substitute case manager when a Japanese-speaking person was needed.[42] And it is only in places where there is a large Asian population, such as San Francisco, that bilingual services in Asian languages are available at all.

In addition, the current flare of anti-immigrant bias in the U.S. has opened another difficult front for Asian Americans. The ban on admitting HIV-infected immigrants to the United States in 1993 angered many Asian and Pacific Islander communities. This ban will particularly affect the estimated 50,000 Filipinos who immigrate to America each year.[43] As early as 1993, the Filipino Task Force on AIDS feared that "the HIV ban on immigration would drive those who are HIV-infected further underground and prevent them from accessing the needed health intervention."[44] Further exacerbating the situation for Californians, voters passed Proposition 187 in 1994, which banned almost all public services to both undocumented immigrants and their American-born children.

As suggested by Ken McLaughlin of the *San Jose Mercury News*, and Jonathan Mann and others, the number of people who are newly infected with HIV will soar in Asia during the next few years, while the rate of new infections will level off in the rest of the world.[45] Thai and Japanese rates of AIDS are already growing dramatically. Simultaneously, economic ties, including sex tourism, between Asia and the U.S. are strong and growing stronger. Clearly immigration bans are not the answer, but education for both new immigrants and residents is crucial.

The five-year period of 1987–92 was one in which Asians and Pacific Islanders in the Bay Area fought to first establish their existence as a community that is susceptible to HIV, then to document the specific risks in a way that acknowledged the diversity of their communities. Simultaneous with the effort to become visible were the struggle for funds, the creative stretch to remold and invent appropriate prevention strategies, and the need to change strategies as the epidemic moved into new age groups and demographic niches.

The first wave of activists and educators established intervention programs for gay and bisexual men and worked with injection drug users; the second wave may continue these programs, while being asked to develop other types of interventions. How the cultural backgrounds of the educators will function when approaching new populations is unclear. The primary activist emphasis of the organizations has been getting resources into their communities and having materials and strategies that are culturally appropriate to various ethnic groups, risk populations, and subcultures (all marked by sexuality, age, gender, and by issues of identification). Differences associated with class, especially with the consequences of poverty, were not as high on the community agenda. Nor was there much concern about women. The former omission may have been due to prioritization of ethnic access "first," so to speak, and a sense that some immigrant communities are still integrated across class lines because of family connections and recent experiences of temporary post-immigration poverty—a condition that may be felt even by the currently wealthy, due to the experience of settling in a new country. Lack of attention to the needs of women can be traced to their lower rates of infection as well as to the dominance of men (all gay or bisexual) in the leadership of the most active organizations.

On the other hand, many of the organizers have suffered exhaustion and "burnout." Several educators commented that doing HIV/AIDS work is exhausting. They put in long, hard hours and never knew if their information was actually being used to prevent AIDS. Some frankly admitted that there was something of a battle between groups due to funds becoming scarce. One educator made the following comment: "People fight about money. It's part of politics . . . it's part of working in AIDS. Personally, I don't relish that." This has caused organizations to "compete as to who provides better services, who has the right to do outreach at certain bars, and who is more equipped," as another noted. The situation is further complicated by the contrast of low rates among Asians in the U.S. with rapidly climbing rates in some parts of Asia, notably Thailand and India.

The lessons of the work of the San Francisco AIDS Foundation indicated that the challenge of providing services for genders, ethnicities, or sexualities different from one's own can be daunting. The competition for funds from new organizations will provide a challenge to existing Asian American AIDS organizations similar to the one faced by the AIDS Foundation. That organization was forced to retreat from its hegemonic AIDS education role in the face of criticism that it was too narrow in its staff and leadership base to provide education for all. While the work of the pioneering Asian American and Pacific Islander agencies may continue, the actual personnel, agencies, and programs will undoubtedly change, perhaps in ways unanticipated or resisted by the early and current activists, as different populations and interest groups begin to gain control of funds and priorities.

When Sex Workers
Run AIDS Organizations[1]

Rates of HIV infection among United States prostitutes are on a par with those of women in the communities of which they are a part. This is because prostitutes often use condoms, even when they have not been specifically educated to do so by AIDS prevention workers. The relatively low rate of sexual transmission (despite the high rates of intravenous drug use among prostitutes) from sex workers to their customers is a function of the procedures that the workers follow as part of their management of sexuality as a business. They routinely use condoms and avoid anal intercourse. The focus of their sexual activity is masturbation and oral sex. In addition, many are adept at applying condoms without the customer's knowledge. Nevertheless, prostitutes are less likely to use condoms with their steadies or lovers than with dates, and those women who are injection drug users or otherwise desperate for money may be convinced to have sex without any protection.

Two different approaches have been taken in response to the potential spread of HIV via prostitution: effective educational strategies combined with testing, on the one hand, and quarantine, on the other. Choosing one or the other has been, in part, a factor of who an agency or governmental entity is trying to protect: the prostitute? the customer? public morality? The decision is also related to the role attributed to prostitution in the spread of HIV. Most people see prostitutes as carriers and transmitters of HIV, although considerable research has indicated that this is not the case.

There is an interesting contradiction in the policy of many state agencies toward prostitution with regard to AIDS: some prostitute education programs run by prostitutes and ex-prostitutes are being funded at the same time that repressive legislation is being passed. The California Prevention Education Project, originally known as the California *Prostitutes* Education Project (Cal-PEP) is a community-based non-profit that fits this model. It is also an organization that has had to contend with permanent tension between acceptability and stigma.[2]

In this chapter, we follow the history of two issues in Cal-PEP. The first is how its leaders managed its stigmatized identity as an organization of "whores and ex-whores." Secondly, we look at the roles of community culture and personal entanglements in determining staff policy and practice. Both types of issues affect many grass roots organizations, especially those in poor communities of color where personal relationships and family connections are often necessary to buffer capitalist exploitation.

In its first phase as a grassroots organization, from 1984 to 1987, Cal-PEP was composed primarily of overworked prostitute advocates and volunteers working on a shoestring budget and providing most services for free. Most of its activities were one-to-one counseling and education, all labor intensive. Community input was high because the organization was run by prostitutes. Its board (advisory at first) and its staff were overlapping and most of the decision-making was by groups, either in the office or at monthly board meetings. However, its leadership for day-to-day decisions was shared by three women: Priscilla Alexander, a white prostitute advocate with strong writing skills; Sharon Kaiser, a white social worker, with sex worker experience; and Gloria Lockett, an African American, who was destined to become the director and the person with whom Cal-PEP is most linked in the public mind.

My own association with the organization included five years as a board member and two as an informal consultant. During this time I interviewed staff, collected documents, and kept sporadic notes.[3] Throughout my association with the organization, and during the preparation of this book, the top leadership of Cal-PEP was aware that I planned to write about them.

In 1987, Cal-PEP moved into a second stage of bureaucratic development, with its incorporation as a non-profit. At this point, it needed to have a real board of directors and an organizational director who were legally "in charge," a structure required by most funding agencies. Gloria Lockett became the official executive director and continues to hold that position as of this writing.

The struggle to have a board that makes decisions plagued Cal-PEP for years, primarily, I believe, because the management of the organization, at least in its early years, was unwilling to relinquish that power to anyone. Cal-PEP's founders felt that they were the people most knowledgeable about the issues of prostitutes, HIV, and street outreach. Another reason that board staffing was difficult for Cal-PEP is that few prostitutes have the ability to sit on the board of a nonprofit. Many of the people that Cal-PEP was reaching were poorly educated, engaged in illegal behavior (drug use and/or prostitution), poor, and in some cases homeless. Despite these problems and very high rates of board turnover, Cal-PEP inched toward a more traditional bureaucracy, finally developing an appropriate cost accounting system and stabilizing both its board and its paid staff in the early 1990s.

Even long after it incorporated, Cal-PEP struggled to maintain its status as a grass-roots advocacy organization. As recently as 1996, Gloria Lockett spoke proudly about her organization in just these terms:

We are respected, we do lots of good work, and we let people know we do good work, and we take care of our clients. We are the people who will fight. When they want a press release or when something is going on that's not right, we put ourselves on the front lines.[4]

At the same time, Lockett is proud of the reputation Cal-PEP has earned for the services it provides. In her own words:

So I think, I know, people *do* respect us. I've gotten letters, we're called all the time. We're called to do trainings, and I've got people that have been with me, you know, seven, eight years, five years. We've got a good team.

We just got another grant to get a state-of-the-art new RV, a 32-footer. And it will actually be a mobile clinic. It will have three HIV counseling rooms, an examination bed in the back, a lab, actually a laboratory with a centrifuge and everything on it, and an awning so that when you want to work in the sun and when it's hot, you can just take it out and put chairs outside. It's going to be wonderful.[5]

Cal-PEP has tried to maintain its grass-roots nature and sense of radical purpose at the same time that it fulfills the requirements of its funders to fit into a bureaucratic capitalist non-profit model. This has inevitably made it suspect in the eyes of the government agencies whose funds it needs. As Lockett puts it:

We are still the people that get targeted a lot, and I think that's because of our background, where we came from. And we don't try to hide where we came from. We're still hiring people that are ex-IV drug users, ex-prostitutes, ex-, you know, homeless people, ex-housewives.

But, I mean, the work that we want to do, and that we cherish doing, is working with what other people call the losers. But to us they're our people. So basically we have moved from being this prostitutes-only organization to being an organization that works with people on the street.

As an organization of and for prostitutes, Cal-PEP had a very difficult time gaining recognition and funding. To understand the legitimation problems of Cal-PEP it is useful to take a side trip to understanding public views of sex workers.

Images of Prostitution

Most of the images evoked by current social constructions of prostitution offend or frighten.[6] The prostitute is at once victim, collaborator, worker, and renegade depending on the context and purpose of her invocation. Each of these socially constructed identities is charged in one way or another and, depending on one's point of view, any of them can elicit negative feelings.[7]

The prostitute as victim is seen as exploited by rapacious pimps, dangerous clients, and the ideological dictates of capitalist patriarchy which produce woman as sexual commodity.[8] In the case of the unrepentant prostitute, the protective status of innocent victim is replaced by the identity of "collaborator." The prostitute as collaborator is the sexist objectification and oppression of all women, particularly if she is unrepentant. The sex worker is then seen as a class traitor to other women by consciously or unconsciously reinforcing the oppressive idea that women are first and foremost sex objects.

Alternatively, the idea of the prostitute as a service worker or professional is well expressed by "Mayflower Madame" Sydney Biddle Barrows. "Are you really doing anything wrong?" she asks rhetorically. "You're getting money that you really need from a man who can certainly afford to part with it. You're providing a real service without hurting or taking advantage of anybody."[9]

Perhaps the darkest vision of the prostitute is as a depraved exploiter of men's sexual needs, charging for that which should be freely given. For those less sympathetic to prostitutes, the image of a woman making money from sex translates into exploitation of the client. The prostitute is then seen as a conniving and lucky cunt getting rich lying on her back and doing only what comes naturally. A California sheriff expressed this sentiment when he said, "You can call them 'sex workers' or anything you want, and it may minimize it in somebody's eyes . . . . But they are charging outrageous prices . . . . It's just a way to make easy money . . . literally thousands of dollars lying on your back . . . . Calling it a 'profession,' that's a bunch of crap."[10]

Equally negative, prostitutes are also thought of as public health menaces. The idea that the prostitute is a pool of contagion (both moral and physical) has a long history. In the eighteenth and nineteenth centuries in Western Europe and the United States, state officials alternately attempted regulation and abolition of prostitution as a means of safeguarding the "public" from venereal disease. In the current era of AIDS, this identification of prostitutes with disease has re-emerged strongly.

In order to arrest rather than just treat those perceived to be disease carriers, the prostitute must be understood to be not only a public health threat but also a law enforcement problem. The justification is that prostitutes threaten the health of the nation's manhood, the purity of its womanhood, and the security of its key building block—the monogamous, heterosexual nuclear family.

While law enforcement tends to justify its fight against prostitution in terms of a defense of family values, some social critics reverse the problem and view these structures of family, gender, and sexuality to be the real source of social ills. For such critics, the prostitute is seen as a potentially subversive social actor. In recent years, this vision of the prostitute has been reclaimed by some feminists as a Bad Girl anti-hero. She is seen as a sexual renegade and a gender outlaw who defies conventional femininity and proper womanhood.

In organizations like Cal-PEP and its parent organization COYOTE (Call Off Your Old Tired Ethics), which were formed to advocate for and provide services to prostitutes, a new and anomalous role has been established—the prostitute as outreach worker or reformed native. Historically, the prostitute often has been seen as an inside informant who can become a convert enlisted to do outreach work to her still-fallen sisters. The interesting and novel aspect of this role in the late twentieth century is that prostitutes increasingly are directing or co-directing their own outreach organizations, not simply being co-opted in some token capacity into existing ones. The AIDS crisis, in particular, has given new life to this redemptive identity of "ex-prostitute." A headline in the *San Francisco Chronicle* announced the work of prostitute-run AIDS organizations in precisely these terms: "Reformed Prostitutes Take to the Streets to Help Their Sisters."[11] The article highlighted the supposed efforts of former prostitutes to "coax women out of the sex trades."

All of these identities combine to produce the "post-modern prostitute," a necessarily fragmented and contradictory identity. Its complexity reveals "prostitution" to be an unstable concept. Within the context of the AIDS epidemic, prostitution as practice, business, and concept has become the social site of constant contestation over meaning and appropriate strategic response.

It is important to note here that prostitutes have never been passive objects in this battle over identity and meaning. At different times and for specific purposes, sex workers have embraced various of these identities and challenged others: WHISPER (Women Hurt in Systems of Prostitution in Revolt) portrays prostitutes as victims; COYOTE projects prostitutes as daring renegades; for the Dutch prostitute's union, the Red Thread, the prostitute is simply a service worker; for Cal-PEP the prostitute is a valuable educational resource for marginalized communities. In other words, sex workers themselves have actively seized on these conflicting identities in competing campaigns for decriminalization, abolition, or legitimation.

The AIDS crisis has provided a powerful avenue for the struggle to legitimize prostitution, especially in countries like the United States where sex work is still a criminal activity. Our government does not view civil rights for sex workers as a legitimate goal for the state to pursue, but it does wish to invest funds in stopping the spread of AIDS. In this context, sex workers may subversively accept the identity of disease carrier in order to secure funding, to force a place at the policy table, and to enhance recognition of their expertise in the public sexual realm.[12]

For sex workers in countries like the Netherlands, where the trade enjoys at least a measure of legality, prostitutes' organizations have tended to focus their attention on protecting sex workers from ill-advised state policies and new regulations rather than attempting to get them out of the trade or into latex.

For most sex workers, condom use during commercial sex is the rule rather than the exception. A serious exception is when workers have little control. Control can be taken away by excessive drug use, coercive clients, or brothel managers who do not allow women to refuse any customer. For this reason, organizations run by sex workers consistently emphasize the need for prostitutes to be professionals ("career prostitutes" versus "drug prostitutes") and to control their working environment. They argue that this kind of workplace control best promotes safer sexual practices. Hansje Verbeek of the Dutch Red Thread notes, "AIDS is not only a ... medical problem, but also primarily a social problem.... The policy on AIDS must become an integral part of the drive to improve the prostitutes' situation. Lifting the ban on brothels ..., consolidating the legal position of prostitutes ... [making them] more independent in doing their work [would be critically important to controlling AIDS]."

This call is echoed by other prostitutes' organizations around the world ostensibly devoted to AIDS outreach work. For example, one of Australia's prostitutes' rights organizations, PROS, has used the AIDS crisis as a means to organize women working in parlors. They provide the women with "condoms, information about STDs, the law and taxation."[13] Similarly, the prostitutes' organization in Thailand, EMPOWER, does much more than AIDS education. It also runs English language classes to help workers better negotiate with clients, counseling services, and workshops on women's rights.

Prostitutes' rights advocate Priscilla Alexander concludes that "Most projects [around the world] have found themselves focusing on more than just the promotion of condoms and safer sexual practices, as they have dealt with problems with police, put pressure on the health care system to provide better services and to treat prostitutes with more respect, and helped the women to establish community-based self-help and self-advocacy organizations."[14]

Becoming Legitimate

Cal-PEP was founded by COYOTE with the help of Project AWARE—an organization at the University of California, San Francisco, funded in 1985 by the CDC to recruit female prostitutes for HIV testing. The history of Cal-PEP's founding and development is the story of a child far outgrowing its parents. By 1993, Cal-PEP had become a community-based non-profit with a $1.4 million budget and thirty-two employees, while both AWARE and COYOTE had shrunk and lost influence.

In the United States, organizing around prostitutes' rights was spearheaded by COYOTE. COYOTE's activism, described in detail by Val Jenness in *Making It Work*, somewhat reduced the deviance and stigma associated with prostitution and improved the legal status of prostitutes, especially in northern California.[15] In spinning off Cal-PEP, COYOTE's leaders saw an opportunity to position the prostitutes' rights movement to receive extensive local, state, and federal funds. They were right, though they may not have foreseen the consequences. For as Cal-PEP grew into a large, well-staffed non-profit, COYOTE struggled along with almost no budget and no staff. For its part, Project AWARE lost its initial contracts with the Centers for Disease Control and was searching for stable funding. How did these changes occur?

COYOTE was founded in the mid-seventies in San Francisco. As an organization of prostitutes and their advocates, it has functioned as a union, a political organization, and a source of member services. COYOTE's political focus has been on decriminalization. Like most prostitutes' rights organizations, it is small. It generally had fewer than twenty active members in the Bay Area. However, its ability to capture the attention of the media led to its imitation in a number of American cities. It has been involved in international networking, especially in Europe, where it has ties with the Red Thread and the Pink Thread of Holland and the prostitutes' unions of France, Germany, and Italy.

By 1985, this San Francisco-based organization had over fifteen years' experience analyzing and fighting the stigmatization and scapegoating of prostitutes. Its relationships with the local sheriff, elements of the press, and local elites were good. It was beginning to respond to the epidemic in a limited way with education programs for its own active members as well as other prostitutes. It had essentially no budget, but several volunteer advocates and members printed flyers, gave talks, and responded to press questions and requests for presentations on AIDS in relation to prostitution.

During this period there was a relatively small national increase in male AIDS cases considered to be caused by transmission from women. Most of these men asserted that the most likely source of infection was sex with a female prostitute. The Centers for Disease Control used these assertions to justify research on prostitutes as potential carriers of HIV. Much of the initial research was designed to map the extent of seropositivity among sex workers. To do the mapping, it was necessary to convince prostitutes to test for the HIV antibody. To talk them into such tests, the projects began to hire prostitutes as outreach workers. (Technically the women were supposed to be *former* prostitutes.) Education was a secondary concern of all of these projects, but ethical and practical considerations led to its incorporation in most of them. One of these projects was Project AWARE at UCSF.

In 1985, Project AWARE turned to COYOTE for help in recruiting female prostitutes for testing. Three employees (two prostitutes and an advocate) were initially paid by the hour for their outreach and education services. These three women gradually came to be defined as experts in AIDS education for prostitutes. They already knew the culture of prostitution, and at Project AWARE they also learned the cultures of AIDS education, funding, and community politics. They were quick learners.

They rapidly became bi-cultural (and in most cases, multi-cultural) experts. Most of the prostitute employees were already socialized into street cultures and ethnic community life. Most had been in jail. And a number were lesbian or bisexual (not uncommon in the world of prostitutes). In fact, they knew a lot about the communities that the researchers were interested in and that the health departments also wanted to reach. COYOTE, as the gatekeeper to the local prostitute population, came to be seen by the AIDS establishment as the best voice of and key to local prostitutes.

COYOTE spun off Cal-PEP as a separate and legally independent organization in 1987. That year, Cal-PEP incorporated and applied for and received its first grant of $50,000 from the California Department of Health Services. Initially, the staff consisted of two ex-prostitutes—who were also working for Project AWARE to do AIDS education in the street with injection drug-using prostitutes.

Cal-PEP's gradual emergence from COYOTE was graphic, bureaucratic, and political. At first the organizations had similar stationery, prepared on the same computer. (See Figure 4.1) For legitimacy, Cal-PEP selected a logo similar to that of COYOTE. It used the same phone number and the same post office box. And even as the agency became a small independent non-profit, they utilized COYOTE's techniques to gain institutional support. They especially drew on manipulation of the public constructions of the prostitute as victim, profession-al, public health menace, renegade, and outreach worker. This appropriation is not surprising, since all the original paid and unpaid employees of Cal-PEP were

Figure 4.1: *Similar stationery of Cal-PEP and COYOTE in 1986.*

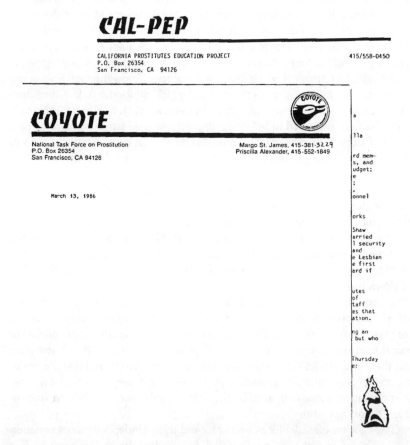

also members of COYOTE. In addition, Cal-PEP leadership managed the public and private funding agencies as if they were tricks (customers): they learned what the funder wanted, negotiated a good payment, warded off the law, and remained aware that their primary loyalty was to each other, not to government agencies, foundations, or any other "straight" group. They were bold about being prostitutes—renegades and educators simultaneously.

By 1988, Cal-PEP was receiving grants not only from DHS, but also from the Centers for Disease Control and the National Institute on Drug Abuse. Then it applied for and received a $350,000 grant from the Robert Wood Johnson Foundation. Cal-PEP was now in competition with other, more mainstream organizations for funds to reach prostitutes. It began to subcontract for AWARE, and AWARE also worked for Cal-PEP as a subcontractor. Cal-PEP had become an active player in the AIDS world.

Eventually, as Cal-PEP began to outgrow both COYOTE and Project AWARE in the area of AIDS prevention for prostitutes, crack users, and other female drug users, it came into conflict with both "parents" and with other competitors in the field of AIDS services.

In 1989, when I first began writing about Cal-PEP, I observed that street identity was still very strong among the three full-time and four part-time staff members. Only gradually had they begun to accept their own legitimacy or appropriateness in the world of health educators, doctors, nurses, and program managers. Only a few years earlier, Cal-PEP's staff had been reluctant even to negotiate with Project AWARE for desks or lockers. One staff member said she was pleased simply to be provided with material; pay was secondary. Another said, "Ho's know how to work out of cars and in the street." To her it was a matter of pride that she did not need a desk or locker. Others were afraid to risk their tentative legitimacy by being seen as too demanding.

By 1991, however, street identity was noticeably weaker, and professional identity was stronger. Though street culture still dominated the style of the organization, both in its outreach techniques and in its management style and its readiness to engage in social conflict, the street identity *per se* was alternately presented and hidden, depending on its strategic usefulness.

In 1989, the presence of an ex-prostitute majority on the board, drawn from the activist ranks of COYOTE, seemed to provide assurance that the organization would continue to play a role in advocacy for prostitutes' rights. By 1991, however, only one COYOTE activist remained on the board, and in 1992 the Cal-PEP board had three men and no COYOTE activists. The rise of Cal-PEP in the AIDS establishment not only diminished COYOTE's standing within the organization, it also undermined the ability of the parent organization to remain viable. The child, as it were, swallowed the parent. Yet without COYOTE, Cal-PEP could never have come into being. In 1989, the most active members of COYOTE were the staff and part of the board of Cal-PEP. In their new roles, they were funded only to do AIDS education. These COYOTE members, as Cal-PEP staff, attended national and international AIDS meetings where they pursued their Cal-PEP agenda—looking for consulting jobs, exchanging information on outreach ideas, and sharing skills and techniques. Only when there was time, or the opportunity to use a stopover on a plane ticket, would they pursue the COYOTE agenda: a broad critique of the way the AIDS epidemic was being managed, the practice of scapegoating, and attempts to regulate sexuality. But over time this small and overworked Cal-PEP staff had less and less time for COYOTE's goals per se.

Conflict between Cal-PEP and COYOTE first became overt in 1990, when COYOTE pressed Cal-PEP to use some of its staff resources and funds to support a conference in San Francisco being organized by COYOTE and the International Committee on Prostitutes' Rights. The organizers, most of whom were friends and colleagues with overlapping membership in each others' groups, including in several cases close connections to, or previous employment in Cal-PEP, expected that Cal-PEP would provide material resources and time to produce the conference. Instead Cal-PEP dragged its organizational feet and eventually refused to do most of the work that the others wanted, citing its funding limitations and its need to keep its spending patterns "clean." The other organizers accused Cal-PEP's leadership of "selling out" to its funders. The conflict was resolved by Cal-PEP management, and the director in particular, who came down on the side of service, "responsibility" to funders, and bureaucratic submission to the terms of its contracts. This decision, which reflected the strategic thinking of its director, helped Cal-PEP to define its autonomy and independence from COYOTE.

Concomitantly, COYOTE members who were not part of the Cal-PEP project grew increasingly distant from those who were. In one interesting development, several of them became active in other AIDS direct-action organizations, such as Mobilization Against AIDS and ACT-UP San Francisco. Their political and sexual radicalism was welcomed in these organizations. Other COYOTE members retired from Cal-PEP, sometimes after considerable public conflict.

One of Cal-PEP's strategies for dealing with the schizophrenia inherent in its attempt to stay true to its origins is explained by Lockett:

> We have two names. One is California Prostitutes Education Project, and the other one is California Prevention Education Project. I try and get everybody just to say "Cal-PEP." I try and sign "Cal-PEP," but some of our funders have been with us a long time, and almost all of our contracts say "California Prostitutes Education Project." But as you know, there are some funders when they see the word "prostitutes," they get real scared, like "Oh no, they're trying to train prostitutes." So if they're conservative, when we write grants, we put "Prevention." If they're not conservative and appreciate the work that we're doing, we say "Prostitutes." We'll probably always have both names.

In the early nineties, Cal-PEP used its original name or its initials. (See Figure 4.2) By 1996, however, California Prevention Education Project was the functional full name of the organization, as seen in figure 4.3.

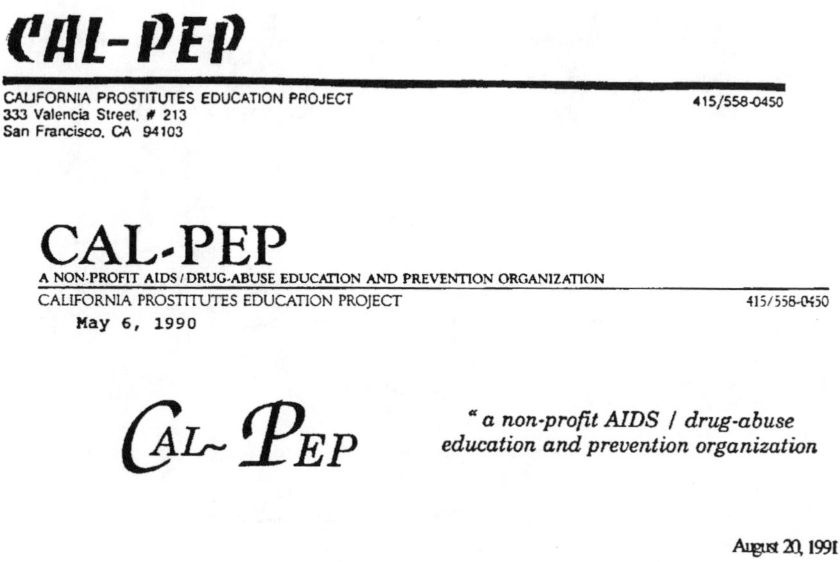

CAL-PEP

CALIFORNIA PROSTITUTES EDUCATION PROJECT
333 Valencia Street, # 213
San Francisco, CA 94103

415/558-0450

CAL-PEP
A NON-PROFIT AIDS / DRUG-ABUSE EDUCATION AND PREVENTION ORGANIZATION

CALIFORNIA PROSTITUTES EDUCATION PROJECT   415/558-0450

May 6, 1990

C̲AL-P̲EP   *" a non-profit AIDS / drug-abuse*
                  education and prevention organization

August 20, 1991

Figure 4.2 *Changing Stationery Masthead for Cal-PEP*

Family Values

Unlike many grassroots AIDS organizations that outgrew their founders, Cal-PEP continues to be stamped by the imprint of its earliest activists. And from the beginning it has also asserted its own values, including familial and community support rather than bureaucratic universalism.

Gloria Lockett, who has led Cal-PEP from its inception, spent her entire adult life, prior to Cal-PEP, working as a prostitute. She never finished high school. In 1981, when she first heard of COYOTE, she was working as the key organizer of an extensive prostitution/call-girl network. Through her involvement with COYOTE she became an early Cal-PEP employee. Soon, as Cal-PEP's first director, not only did she lead the organization in extensive growth, she also turned to her past associates to join her staff. She hired the woman who had handled the books for the prostitution network as the financial director of Cal-PEP. The man who was previously their contact with the police and lawyers and who recruited new prostitutes (the person some would call a pimp) became the volunteer personnel director. By 1993, he was also chair of the board of directors.

These three organizational leaders, all African American, believed in what I would term "family and community" values. It is part of their system of values that they support the prostitution "family" in which they worked for many years

NAME_____   AGE____   DATE_____

CAL-PEP CALIFORNIA PREVENTION AND EDUCATION PROJECT

SEXUALLY TRANSMITTED DISEASE
PRE-TEST

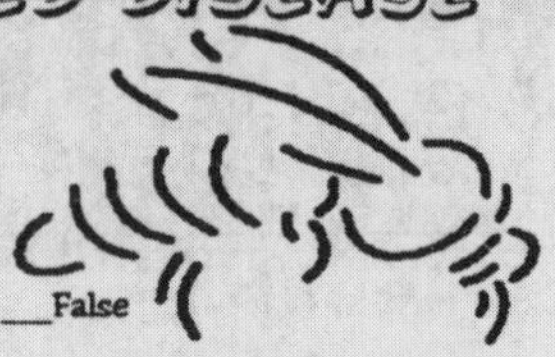

1) Herpes is spread by direct Skin to Skin contact. ___True or ___False

2) What does your body create to fight off viruses?
   a. Anti-Heroes   c. Anti-Bodies
   b. Hard Bodies   d. Anti-Pasto

3) Syphilis, Trichomonias, Gonorrhea and Chlamydia are some Bacteria that can be cured with Anti-Biotics   ___True or ___False

4) Untreated Syphilis can lead to blindness, Heart Disease, and Brain Damage.
   ___True or ___False

5) Anytime someone gets a STD they will get a Burn, Itch or a Drip.   ___True or ___False

6) Most STD's are not as serious for women.   ___True or ___False

7) HPV (Genital Warts) often have to be burned or frozen off by a doctor.   ___True or ___False

8) What is Pelvic Inflammatory Disease?
   a. Random and uncontrollable erections
   b. A big gut
   c. A serious genital tract infection for women

9) In the US about how many "clap" (Gonorrhea) cases occur yearly?
   a. 20,000   b. 1.4 Million   c. 500,000

10) The only place to get STD treatment is at Government clinics. ___True or ___False

11) STD's have no connection to HIV transmission. ___True or ___False

12) Many STD's can make you sterile.   ___True or ___False

PROTECT THE BLOOD!
NAME_____

Figure 4.3 *Cal-PEP identifies itself as the California Prevention and Education Project in 1993 Materials.*

and which continues to provide them with a supportive social network. They also prioritize African American concerns.

As it grew, Cal-PEP was attacked, especially by some of its competitors, ostensibly for replicating the staff, the management style, and the structure of their previous network of prostitutes, an organization that was, after all, illegal. Although the ostensible charge was nepotism, an implication that these leaders carried an essential and inescapable criminality adhered to these attacks. In contrast, when other non-profit directors hire their work associates from, say, a bank or another agency where they had once worked together, no such complaints are heard unless the individuals are clearly incompetent. The difference is that Cal-PEP's leading staffperson was an assertive, street-savvy African American prostitute, an identity practically guaranteed to cause anxiety in a white middle-class bureaucrat—especially one who hears that his or her money is in the hands of such a woman. Interestingly, Cal-PEP's pro-prostitution values have also caused conflict with some feminists, both white and black, who initially supported the organization. For example, several feminists left the board because they believed that the man who was helping manage the organization had too much power and that the women who were ostensibly in charge were not making the decisions.

The assertion of familial values also caused the organization some serious problems of public perception and on-going funding crises. In 1993, the external world crashed down on Cal-PEP when a series of exposé articles appeared on the front pages of the major Bay Area dailies.[16] I was involved with Cal-PEP at the time as a board member, as well as an observing sociologist. The following extensive excerpt from my field notes of August 31, 1993 gives the flavor and intensity of this period.

I had seen two articles in the *San Francisco Examiner* on Cal-PEP . . . concerning allegations about Ralph, Freddie, Gloria, and their connections in both the past and the present. Main emphases: Ralph as pimp, Freddie as his wife, Ralph as chair of the board of Cal-PEP, Freddie and Gloria getting too much money. Etc. I was quoted in the article, one of the few nice comments.

Gloria and I met for a walk around the lake. She told me in passing, near the end of the walk, that she had been spending long hours at the gym and trying to walk every day to reduce stress. Last Sat. she spent all day at the gym, but was still tense when she got home.

She described her problems:
Ralph has resigned as chair of the board, but does not really want to resign from the board overall. He also tells her that this is white people trying to destroy the organization. He wants her to hold fast (resist racism). Also, he believes that she won't get other people to work as hard as him—or he tells her this.

Doris Butler [an African American woman with AIDS featured in the film *Absolutely Positive*] agreed to be chair of the board but has told Gloria that she thinks she can't do it as long as Ralph is still on the board, and that he won't let her really "be" chair but will continue to try to run things.

Our conversation goes back and forth with her telling me the problems and my asking questions, giving my opinions, advice. Sometimes I think to myself: Nancy, do you have the right to do this? What does it mean to say these things, to "interfere" with your own opinion? She doesn't have to listen, but I think she does.

First we talk about Ralph. I agree with Doris Butler that he should be dropped as chair and also side with Doris on his leaving the board. Gloria talks about the fact that no one has done anything illegal, but this is the perception. At a meeting she went to, people reminded her that all black people hire "family," and she adds, other people as well do it too. So is it really necessary for her, for Cal-PEP, to have Ralph go?

My main thrust is that the perception is a problem and, if it were just perception, that would be something to handle and might not require so much change, but it is also an objective problem because she can't get Freddie to act right, partly on account of Ralph, i.e., Freddie goes to Ralph instead of to Gloria.

Gloria says that if she makes Ralph resign from the board and fires or does something about Freddie, this will be very hard on her home life. I tell her she has a choice: She can resign from Cal-PEP. "NO!" I also reinforce the idea that she has a specific responsibility to the organization and that is separate from her responsibility and loyalty to the family. You can hire your family if they can do the job, but if they can't you have to let them go. She says she did this with her daughter and others. So you have to do it here, I say.

She thanks me etc. I encourage her to talk with someone from the Support Center [a technical assistance organization for non-profits] about the crisis and get structural suggestions. I also tell her I will help with hiring someone for Freddie's replacement if she would like. When we part I am thinking, should I offer to be on the board again for a while? . . . although I don't really want to. (I don't.)

I also remind her that everyone believes in her. (She has individual charisma, which repeatedly survives any attacks on the organization.) And that the system of funding and funders has no ethics, it just moves on. If she and Cal-PEP don't get it together, they will just give the money to someone else who may not do the same job as Cal-PEP would but will do something. It's her call.

We stop and get a sandwich, and then she drives back from the lake to her office and my car. I tell her that I know she will do the right thing. I feel I should do more, but I'm not ready to know yet what it is.[17]

A few months later, the man of the family resigned from the Cal-PEP board and ended his role as volunteer personnel director as well. While Cal-PEP lost one contract due to the scandal, it retained all the others and was able to survive with its employee roster intact. In the following years its leaders gradually rebuilt the organization into a new family, this time one of outreach workers and office staff, still headed by the charismatic (maternal) leadership of the initial director. The organization has parties and attends to its internal relationships. In fact, in its own form, we could see it as a female-centered, semi-communal bureaucracy.

Like many other community-based organizations that began as movements for social change, Cal-PEP discovered that in order to survive in a capitalist non-profit environment, it had to find some way to conform to non-profit corporate norms. Despite its commitment to its family and community, Cal-PEP consciously tried to follow the standard bureaucratizing path, moving from a grassroots phase, through a transitional incorporation phase, to a third level, full-scale bureaucracy. Lockett and others understood growth and legitimation as primary paths to programmatic and financial success. They were aware that funding by mainstream foundations and by government agencies required a particular organizational form. So Cal-PEP made the necessary changes but retained as much as possible of the flavor of past and daily lives.

Although Cal-PEP has had annual budgets of over $700,000 for several years, it is not yet a professionalized bureaucracy. Unlike some other large AIDS organizations, it still specializes in face-to-face community and street outreach. Its staff gives trainings, but they do not specialize in them or in the provision of materials to other organizations who do the same sort of outreach that Cal-PEP does. Additionally, the organization continues to use community workers, such as addicts in recovery and ex-sex workers, as opposed to the professionally trained. Its work is not capital intensive and it does not charge for services. On the other hand, Cal-PEP continues to recruit more elite board members. Like organizations that are of more "legitimate" birth, Cal-PEP must be especially attentive to the political world in order to protect itself and its clients, so that work can go ahead. Consequently, there is always at least one politician's aide on the board.

Over the years, Cal-PEP was successful in a number of competitive funding situations because it could present itself as the only legitimate voice in its urban area (and one of very few nationally) for African American women and men who make their living on the street by trading body services for sustenance. Cal-PEP is increasingly extending its claim to represent a wider and wider range of poor men, women, and teenagers in African American communities who are simultaneously struggling with issues of poverty, drugs, and sexuality, even in those cases where sex is not "sold." The object of this new framing is to provide Cal-PEP with a broader mandate for more governmental and foundation funding, which in turn will further institutionalize and legitimate the organization. This will then enable it to do more "survival" work, about which its members are quite fervent.

No matter how broadly Cal-PEP stretches its mandate, it distinguishes itself from other competing organizations in claiming an identity rooted in prostitution, poverty, and street life. But the legitimation of the organization under these terms does not automatically translate into legitimation for prostitutes or advancement of their rights. As Gloria Lockett wearily noted,

> The fact is, we are ex-prostitutes .... Somebody made a statement not too long ago calling us "Cal-WHORES" instead of Cal-PEP. It gives me headaches to make sure that I do things right all the time because of my background. I know people are watching me. I know people want us to mess up ... either for being black or for being a prostitute or for being a woman, or for all three of those.[18]

For prostitutes organizing for greater legitimacy in the 1990s, contestations over identity remain core concerns. In the midst of the AIDS crisis, the prostitute is still likely to be defined as some combination of victim and menace, particularly a public health menace. Prostitutes have not only resisted but also manipulated this fear of the diseased sex worker.

While Cal-PEP and similar AIDS-related organizations may be limited in their ability to challenge the stigmatization of prostitutes as diseased (and indeed may be partially reinforcing that identity), ironically, their stigmatized status may give them legitimacy among the population they are most interested in reaching. Despite its idiosyncrasies in the eyes of white public health professionals and bureaucrats, Cal-PEP continues to receive public funding not only because its organizers are effective, but also because they can politically represent a constituency that funders must address.

Pushing the Point:
Anarchism, Genocide,
and Needle Exchange

As I write about needle exchange, I think of my friend Helen who has Type I diabetes and needs to inject insulin daily. She has been without her own pancreatic production of insulin since she was nineteen. At one point in the past, she injected insulin less frequently, but now she uses "tight control." This involves monitoring her blood three to four times daily (by sticking her finger, dropping blood on a test strip and slipping the strip into a meter, then waiting thirty seconds for a reading on her sugar level) and injecting insulin—on rising, eating, and before going to sleep.

In her bathroom are two Sharps disposal buckets with syringe tops sticking out. On a small bathroom chest a syringe and two insulin bottles rest, casually interspersed with a hair brush, a wash cloth, and *Third Force* magazine. The refrigerator has more insulin. At my house, she has left syringes in the bathroom drawers and insulin in the refrigerator, just in case. When we are at a restaurant, and there is some privacy, Helen might turn her back to the nearest patrons, slip out her syringe and load the insulin. Then she will lift up her shirt, pull down the waistband of her jeans a little and gently inject on the side of her abdomen. The syringe is recapped and back in her pocket in less than a minute.

I think about what Helen's life would be like if diabetes was not medicalized as a disease. Suppose it were just a condition of life, like the increasing farsightedness of old age or aching feet or bad posture? Suppose her treatment of it were considered a matter of choice or a personal attempt to make her life different than her natural lot? Even if her activity were still legal but not defined as a medical necessity, there would be no insurance to pay for insulin, syringes, and blood glucose monitoring equipment. She would have to pay full cost, somewhere in the range of $150-$200 a month just for supplies.

And if she were poor and could not pay, what might she do? She would not be able to buy all the syringes, insulin, or test strips she needed. What would she skimp on? Insulin? Test strips? Doctors' visits? Needles? Perhaps she would inject less often or use less insulin and watch her body deteriorate. Would she then deny that her health was getting worse. Or steal what she needed?

What if the insulin itself were illegal? What if her possession of syringes was criminal? She would have to buy her insulin on the black market, also her needles and syringes. Her kit would no longer be just a "kit"; it would become her "works," her illegal "paraphernalia." If she did not want to steal or buy on the black market, she would have to borrow needles from other users. What would she do as the ones she had got dull? Sharpen them? What about cleaning? What if she were out and had nowhere to clean her syringes, to do her boiling and bleaching, or else risk the possibility of hepatitis or HIV?

The simple and complete reason that there is no HIV epidemic among diabetics equivalent to that among "illicit" users is that diabetic needle use is both legal and covered by insurance, (which Helen is fortunate enough to have). Self-management of insulin-dependent diabetes is not illegal, but by imagining such a scenario we can understand the structure and consequences of the illegality of injection drug use without having to confront an already constructed set of judgments about mood-altering injectables. This stripped-down focus on the consequences of criminalization of needle use allows us to see needle users as rational people with needs. It may also help us understand the ethical motivation of needle exchange activists.

The illogical and stigmatizing ways that even those who are presumably at the center of HIV and substance abuse policy think about injection drug users was brought home to me by an article in the *New York Times* on September 20, 1995. A front-page article reported on the important findings by a panel of the National Academy of Sciences that needle exchange programs reduce HIV infection. A sidebar addressed the notion that drug users share needles as a bonding ritual. The sidebar article gave credit to anthropologist Steven Koester for proving to the Centers for Disease Control that "sharing [needles] was an act of desperation" not a bonding ritual.[1] According to T. Stephen Jones, of the HIV/AIDS prevention program of the Centers for Disease Control, the bonding notion had its origins in a study done in the Haight Ashbury district of San Francisco in the early 1970s. The notion of bonding had been used as a partial excuse by the federal government since the late 1980s for not supporting needle exchange or distribution programs. It seems that people at the CDC believed (or said they believed) that even if you gave junkies clean needles they would still share.

Koester's field work demonstrated that anti-paraphernalia laws and the illegality of various drugs made it too risky for users to carry syringes or dope. In Denver, according to Koester, users went to shooting galleries where they could find privacy (safety) and a needle, even if the needles were sometimes contaminated, blunted, or less effective than new ones.

Jones heard of Koester's work and invited him to the CDC. "His conclusions and similar findings by other investigators dispelled the assumption that needle-sharing was a bonding rite but was something forced on them by circumstances . . . ."[2]

Why would someone use a dirty, beaten-up needle when she could use a clean, sharp one? Only if there were something odd and irrational in her behavior. It is this stigmatization and "othering" that is really behind the "bonding" theory. The stigmatization of the intravenous drug user as an "addict" with a disease that is mental as well as physical was the 1970s contribution of social science to the debate over the legality of mood-altering substances. The earlier judgment was re-assessed in 1995 by a comparable set of scientists—the anthropologist and the epidemiologist, who now declare the earlier judgement suspect. "What do you know?" they intone. "These 'criminals' are acting rationally given the illegality of their situation."

But even if faith in federal assessments of scientific knowledge leads us to accept that in 1994 (when the National Academy of Sciences panel began its work) the CDC and the federal government needed more data to decide on the appropriateness of funding needle exchange, evidence of the drug users' attempts to protect themselves from HIV had already been published almost a decade earlier.

In 1985, Don Des Jarlais, Samuel Friedman, and William Hopkins reported on the changing behavior of intravenous drug users in New York City once they became aware of the risk of AIDS through infected needles. In the late spring of 1983, news of and concern about the epidemic filtered into the authors' Street Research Unit, an ethnographic storefront operation in a high-use area. By the fall, via interviews with eighteen intravenous drug users who were not in treatment, they found that all knew about the epidemic and believed that AIDS was spread through the sharing of needles.

> They [the users] also reported an increased demand for "new" needles among intravenous drug users as a result of AIDS . . . . One indication that the demand for new needles had been sustained came in the summer and fall of 1984, when we heard reports of the selling of "resealed" needles. Needle sellers were placing used needles back into the original packaging, resealing the packaging, and then selling the needle as new. The resealing is done with heat sealing machines that can be purchased in local hardware stores . . . . To study the demand for new needles in greater depth, our Street Research Unit conducted interviews with persons "hawking" needles on the street during the spring of 1985 . . . . Eighteen of twenty-two (eighty-two percent) needle sellers reported that new needle sales had increased over the last year . . . . One seller was chanting "Get the good needles, don't get the bad AIDS" as a sales pitch for his wares.[3]

The researchers concluded that the "data clearly contradict the stereotype of intravenous drug users as incapable of modifying their behavior and as unconcerned with their health." This report was published in 1985 in *Annals of Internal Medicine*, one of the most distinguished medical journals in the U.S. It was followed by other studies that provided similar results.

In 1987, Friedman and his colleagues reported on even more extensive behavioral adjustments to the epidemic in their New York City neighborhood. They began to talk of "self-organizing" as a way of comparing the attempts by users to protect themselves with the more successful attempts by the gay community. They noted serious obstacles to organizing by injection drug users on the individual level: Addiction takes time and energy and poverty limits access to resources. They also noted obstacles at the level of local organization and culture: The predatory social relationships of the drug market result in distrust and a lack of solidarity. On a broader societal level, severe legal repression and stigma, including a hostile press and public, raise serious barriers to organizing.

On the other hand, the researchers found examples of organizing by current and former users including a New York group, ADAPT, which was made up of ex-users and adopted a nonjudgmental attitude toward existing users.[4] But the most striking organizations were the *junkiebonds* of the Netherlands; these organizations of injection drug users began before the HIV epidemic to combat the spread of hepatitis among needle users and were now continuing with specific grassroots anti-AIDS strategies.

Friedman's interest in social movements and community organizing kept the National Drug Research Institute research teams focused on the actual behavior and potential of the users.[5] His own and his colleagues' articles on drug users' responses to AIDS were published shortly before needle exchanges burst onto the American scene, first in Tacoma, Washington, in early 1988. Needle exchange programs to combat AIDS were established as early as 1986 in England and Scotland, where pharmacists were also being encouraged, but not required, to sell needles for "non-therapeutic" purposes, i.e., to drug users.[6]

In other words, a new discourse and a new set of social institutions concerning injection drug users and ways of cooperating with their own attempts to protect themselves from HIV were developing. Despite the limitations imposed by stigmatization and criminality, these changes paralleled the new organizations and institutions developing for AIDS prevention among gay men, prostitutes, and people of color. Each group was confronting a set of stigmas, stereotypes, moral condemnations, and legal issues and developing a language that justified its activity on the grounds that the epidemic's deadliness required the larger society to "bracket" its judgments and allow the members of the group to stay alive by protecting themselves from the virus. After all, the representatives were arguing, even if drug use is illegal, the state has not mandated a death sentence as the penalty for shooting up.

In San Francisco, one such needle exchange organization, Prevention Point, has been in operation since 1988. By 1996, services were being provided four evenings a week for two hours at ten stationary locations in areas of the city with sizable needle using populations. These are all multi-ethnic, low-income neighborhoods.

Like most other needle exchanges, Prevention Point participants exchange needles rather than merely receive new sterile ones. This requirement is intended to reduce the number of contaminated syringes in circulation. Outreach workers also provide information on safer sex and drug use, referrals to drug treatment programs and health care agencies, and tangible items such as bleach, alcohol wipes, cottons, and condoms. Program providers act as conduits to such other social services as drug counseling and referrals to drug treatment programs, health care services, and HIV-related services.

Prevention Point began as an act of civil disobedience by a group of pagan, hippie anarchists who wanted to force the state to provide clean needles to the criminalized injection drug users of California.[7] Throughout the following account, we will see that Prevention Point's anarchism has produced a unique situation: It has survived for eight years as a large group of decentralized volunteers who do the work of exchanging needles; but their material goods (needles, bleach, cotton, AIDS prevention guides), and to some extent even the sites where they work, are now "managed" by a small hierarchically organized staff who publicly represent the needle exchange and over whom the volunteers have no effective control.

Luis Kemnitzer, a long-time volunteer, describes the start of Prevention Point this way:

> There was research going on about risk of injection drug use. Also, people were doing HIV testing of the drug users. They immediately realized that they had to give the results to the people tested. That led to having counseling, because you couldn't give the results back, especially if the results were positive, without providing counseling.
>
> This then led to the realization that maybe you could do something to slow infection rates beyond counseling and that was to clean up the needles somehow. So first, people realized that you could distribute bleach.
>
> Jennifer [Lorvick], at Urban Health Study [a San Francisco-based drug research organization], was the first person to actually figure out the mechanics. She put the bleach in little bottles. Then they [UHS] started distributing condoms and bleach. Nevertheless, they got in trouble with the cops, or I should say the recipients got in trouble with the cops. Especially the women got in trouble about the condoms because they were treated as a sign of prostitution, and the woman could be harassed or arrested for having a lot of them. Also, police are rumored to have punched needle holes in the condoms. But with publicity, eventually people were able to slow that up and get the police department to stop it.
>
> But workers realized that this distribution was not enough because it is a problem to get clean needles, so they thought it would be a responsibility of theirs to somehow get clean needles to the users. On the one side there was responsibility and commitment. On the other side, there were the police.
>
> Meanwhile there were some pagan anarchist cd [civil disobedience] hippie junkies who wanted to do something about this. This last group, including Moher Downing and Rose Dietrich, were the founders of Prevention Point.
>
> They brought in the non-hierarchical model. They planned to get arrested from the start in order to get the issue into the public eye. Once they were arrested they planned to move on to getting various celebrities arrested as a way to draw attention and then change the law.

However, they did not get arrested. And that missed arrest led to the long-term organization of Prevention Point, including its transformation from a civil dis-

obedience organization—of an unusual nature—to a somewhat anarchic network of small "service" organizations.

What were the nuts and bolts as well as the original intent of this initially illegal activity? In August 1988, the founders-to-be of Prevention Point began meeting. The group consisted of fewer than ten women and men who shared some
important characteristics. Everyone had some experience using mood-altering
drugs. All were involved in AIDS prevention work or research with injection drug
users. All had experience with civil disobedience in the anti-nuclear movement of
the 1980s, and all but one identified as anarchist and pagan.

These origins in anarchism and paganism are significant in terms of both the
culture of Prevention Point and the organizational forms its leaders chose. From
the start, as Kemnitzer noted, they expected to be arrested, but they did not want
users to face arrest. They did not know about the Tacoma exchange, begun in
August, although they were aware of and in fact had helped develop the bleach
distribution projects in San Francisco. Although they did not use the language of
"harm reduction"—a public health philosophy that advocates doing what is possible within a potentially dangerous social context to reduce harm, even if one
cannot remove the entire threat—they were operating within this prevention
model. The organizers knew they wanted to have an "anonymous, non-judgmental, user-friendly model with no requirements for participation other than the
possession of a syringe and the willingness to exchange."[8]

In order to design a procedure that would meet these criteria the organizers,
in good action-research tradition,[9] arranged a hot dog dinner for needle users
living at the Ambassador, a single-room occupancy hotel in San Francisco's Tenderloin district. They walked the halls, knocking on doors, telling people of the
available hot food, and handing out a flyer that proclaimed:

> We are a group of concerned folks not associated with any organization. We are tired
> of waiting for the needle laws to change. We are willing to be arrested in order to make
> clean needles available to people who need them. We would like to start a "peoples' nee-
> dle exchange program." Each week we would come to the Tenderloin for about two
> hours and exchange one dirty needle for one clean one. This may seem unfair, but we
> want to duplicate the kind of program that we believe could be made law here in
> California. Only a needle exchange [as opposed to simple distribution] seems to fit that
> bill.

The flyer went on to talk about general plans and ask for feedback. The organizers asked each person arriving for supper where it would be best to set up the
needle exchange and how to organize it. Within a few days they went to the various locations suggested to further examine their potential. The organizers consciously adopted four criteria in selecting sites: the ability to mimic street syringe
selling, including surreptitious transactions; accessibility and convenience for
intravenous drug users; no infringement on existing social interactions, legal or
illegal; and sufficient space to locate monitors who could alert participants to
potential problems with police or local merchants.

After some research, the organizers chose an approach that used a "stationary team" and a "roving team." The stationary team was located near a park where intravenous drug users frequently congregated. Prevention Point assumed that workers at this site would be arrested by the police because of the site's visibility. Initially it was considered a decoy to deflect attention from the mobile part of the distribution system, which was designed for both safety and to reach those who would not come to the more open site for fear of identification or arrest.

On October 28, 1988, the organizers had their final preparatory meeting. The agenda included such matters as a needle supply report, role plays, legal issues, and how to handle the media if there were arrests. They prepared an informed consent script for those who came to get needles that warned them the exchange might be illegal.

The first day of the exchange, November 2, was the Day of the Dead, a date specifically chosen by the organizers both to commemorate those who had died from AIDS and because of its pagan origins. In its own history of that night, which Prevention Point has been able to make official by setting up its own "Prevention Point Research Team" (indistinguishable in membership from the organization's core members and their partners), thirteen Prevention Point members exchanged thirteen needles in a two-hour period in the Tenderloin.[10] The numbers may be mythical, but they do have a recognizable pagan significance and are therefore an important part of the organization's origin story.

After the distribution, the Prevention Point founders gathered for the first of their post-distribution meetings to discuss the process and make plans for the future. The agenda included the need for money, planning for the next exchange (the following week), and ideas for combining disposal of needles with the still-anticipated arrests.

When no arrests followed, Prevention Point settled in for the longer struggle to change public policy. They continued the exchange, began to build community support both for the exchange per se and for an anticipated "coming out" in the press, and they began to strategize about ways to influence local and state policy. Almost a year later, Prevention Point delivered 2,000 used needles to a San Francisco Health Commission hearing considering legalizing needle exchanges. Between November, 1988, and that hearing in September, 1989, Prevention Point had exchanged more than 100,000 needles. By 1992 it had become the most extensive exchange in the country, having exchanged over one million needles at five San Francisco sites.[11]

From the start Prevention Point was concerned about its image in the press. Organizers wanted to show that their model was appropriate to the situation and did not want to be dismissed because of their organizational style, personal and cultural commitments, or politics, all of which were alternative. Unlike ACT-UP, for example, which strove to assert its cultural identity as part of its politics of change, Prevention Point wanted to hide its identity from the mainstream while at the same time revealing certain aspects of itself to its user-participants— sympathy to and solidarity with drug users, willingness to risk arrest, and anarchist leanings. One of the organization's internal handouts illustrates both their approach and their sense of humor:

Things we will not say to the media
(a working list)

1. We won't reveal names of people involved, location(s) of the exchange, or nights that the exchange operates. We will say that it operates in "an area of high IV drug use several times a week."
2. We won't say the names of researchers involved in the evaluation.
3. We won't talk about outfit girl or tell the story about the old lady kicking the baby carriage.
4. We won't ever admit to distributing a needle without exchanging it.
5. We won't say where we get our funding though we will say we are supported by "private contributions."
6. We won't say that we have been given pens, buttons, dice, plungers, bags of marijuana, etc., in lieu of used syringes.
7. We won't say that we had one stolen.
8. We won't say where we get our needles although we will say that "we are buying them and not diverting them."
9. We will not xerox or circulate this list.
10. Do not reveal our political leanings, such as anarchism, paganism.[12]

As winter wore on, Prevention Point members began practicing for their coming out in the media, planned for March 1989, when a Mayoral Task Force was due to make some pronouncements on needle exchange. They consciously picked two "poster girls" as interviewees, both of whom were willing to be photographed and named—Tia Wagner, an African American, and Rose Dietrich, a white woman. They discovered that a reporter for the *San Francisco Chronicle* was about to publish a story on the exchange and decided to cooperate, giving their first interviews. The front-page story appeared on March 13, 1989, and began the public career of Prevention Point.[13] Within a week the head of the Department of Public Health urged that needle exchange be considered for the city,[14] and one arrest of a Prevention Point volunteer occurred.[15] The charges were dropped, and the moves toward legalization and funding of the exchange continued.

Between the time of the Mayoral Task Force Report, which recommended needle exchange as possibly "beneficial in curtailing the spread of AIDS in the IDU population," and a fall hearing before the city's Health Commission, which would have to authorize such a program, various individuals and community organizations responded to needle exchange. The idea very quickly became racially politicized when significant opposition was voiced by Naomi Gray, an African American member of the Commission. She argued against the proposal because it encouraged illegal behavior for which African Americans were more likely than whites to be arrested and sentenced. There was no evidence that it was effective, she claimed, and it sent the wrong message to youth: "that it's OK to break the law if there is a slight possibility that it would protect them against AIDS." Needle exchange was also opposed by the majority of black religious leaders and their followers. Gray concluded her written statement with these words:

> Imposing a program on a people who are against it will not work politically or other-
> wise and will create a divisive debate here and in Sacramento over the legality of a plan
> to distribute clean needles. These energies could be better spent fighting for more edu-
> cation, prevention and treatment funds to fight AIDS and crack cocaine. This would be
> a more productive outcome.[16]

In response, Prevention Point, a predominantly white organization, drew on its multiracial community support, including the Third World AIDS Advisory Task Force, the Latino Coalition on AIDS/SIDA, and the Black Coalition on AIDS, all of which were very supportive of the needle exchange program. In addition to its public support of Prevention Point, the Latino Coalition had sponsored a needle exchange site with Prevention Point in the Mission district of the city.

Charges of racial genocide and assertions that whites were imposing foreign and unwanted solutions on black communities have been prominent in a number of cities where needle exchange has been attempted. In New York, for example, African American opposition to needle exchange programs was widespread in 1987 and 1988, when that city was attempting to establish an experimental program. In January of 1988, when ADAPT received widespread publicity about a planned distribution to addicts, the city cut off its funding for three months. When the Department of Health did start a limited exchange program in November of 1988, racial criticism was voiced by New York Mayor David Dinkins, the chair of the City Council's Black and Hispanic Caucus, Congressman Charles Rangel, the head of another drug treatment program, and several prominent clergy.

Some of these black leaders felt that the exchanges would keep the black community endlessly chained to drugs. Others thought that it was tantamount to abetting the crime of drug abuse. One flatly stated, "I am not in favor of cooperating with evil."[17] As a result of black opposition in New York, the health department's needle exchange program was severely curtailed. It operated out of a health clinic near a police station and far away from the nearest location frequented by injection drug users. The combination of government sponsorship and location may have doomed the New York program to low levels of exchange from the start.[18] The Department of Health exchange was later supplemented with less institutionally based services, but the 1988 New York experience was very much on the minds of San Franciscan needle exchange proponents throughout 1989.

In Boston, in 1990, Jon Parker, a white activist, had set up a branch of his National AIDS Brigade needle exchange project in an African American neighborhood without working with community people. The ensuing debacle led to physical confrontations, picketing, and the closing of the Boston needle exchange program.[19]

Memos from Prevention Point's files and research conducted by the Institute for Scientific Analysis indicate that the issue of racial representation continued to nag the organization. In a media worksheet from February 1989, the "racial issue" appeared in a list of "hard questions" that might be asked by the press. The topic listed was "whether they were participating in genocide through promotion of IDU in minority communities." In other words, was Prevention Point putting guns in the hands of members of the minority community by providing users with needles and making it easier for them to shoot up? Yet another question to be answered, and a difficult one, as Prevention Point would learn. The organization began as predominantly white and has continued to be predominantly white in its volunteer base. As late as 1995, when it had expanded to twelve sites at eight locations, 70 percent of its volunteer "staff" was white.[20] In 1989, at the time of the initial development of Prevention Point, the injection drug-using population in San Francisco was estimated at approximately 49 percent white, 26 percent Latino, and 24 percent African American. Ethnicity of users of the Prevention Point services was approximately 51 percent white, 31 percent African American, 12 percent Latino, 3 percent Native American, and 3 percent Asian.[21]

By 1990 the race issue was clearly on the table, as minutes from a Prevention Point retreat demonstrated. Half the discussion was about making sure that the Prevention Point teams were multi-cultural and reflective of the specific composition of the neighborhoods in which they worked. The minutes summarized concerns:

> Needle exchange must be street-based and sensitive and responsible; no suits—blend in—not just clothing or complexion, but attitude, sensitivity, hipness, comfort to MIRROR THE CLIENTELE according to the NEIGHBORHOOD; this reduces judgmental stuff and makes it accessible; cultural/class affinity; ability to hang. A model: The aggregate of all the neighborhood teams reflects multi-cultural and multi-racial representation, but teams should be organic and appropriate to their neighborhoods including language. E.g. Native Americans in the Mission, signers everywhere, blacks from Bayview on a Bayview team, a primarily Japanese team for around Japantown.[22]

Despite (or perhaps because of) its white, hippie, anarchist, pagan origins, Prevention Point did become the most successful of the needle exchanges. Building community support and attention to neighborhood politics were the primary sources of its success.

In February 1994, two relatively new white volunteers, Alex Kral and Charles Pearson, decided to start an exchange site in a predominantly black and poor area of the city. According to Kral,

> There was a large amount of people that weren't using needle exchange that lived in that area right over there. So I said, "Well, this is perfect. I think that's where we should

do it." And I went and talked to some outreach workers, and the outreach workers basically said, "Yeah, that those projects right there, there's probably fifty or sixty injection drug users who live there, and they aren't being served. We've been wanting to try to do this for years now in this neighborhood." And so consequently we decided to set one up there. And the process by which we did that was basically we talked to all the people, we went to the Western Addition Neighborhood Association meeting. We went to the tenant's association at those projects, we went to the cops in Northern Station, we went to the three kind of most well-known church leaders in the Fillmore, and we went to Ella Hutch Community Center. And we talked to all the leaders there and kind of asked about their concerns and thoughts and everything like that, and in that way kind of got the whole neighborhood rallied around it and made sure that we would take care of all the concerns of people in the neighborhood.[23]

To assist them, Kral and Pearson had help from two African American outreach workers. One had been working in the neighborhood for fifteen years. Two more African American men from the neighborhood already active in AIDS work joined them. But it was Kral and Pearson who went to the meetings and generated public support from the community.

People were pleased, and they didn't play the race cards at all. We were expecting them, but there wasn't really the concern. And when we started the site, the first day of the site we had the two [African American] outreach workers kind of roaming all of the site for a couple of hours before and trying to get people involved and this and that, people to come out. And then we had the four of us, which were the two of us, Charles and I, white, and then two other African American people. And actually after about a month or so, the other people quit because they moved across the Bay so they didn't have time to do it. So we only had the outreach workers for the first two weeks actually, to kind of, and I think they helped a lot in legitimizing us as people to the community, though we only saw about thirteen or fourteen people those first two times.

Throughout its history Prevention Point has been able to cross the color line in multi-racial neighborhoods because of this type of groundwork and nonjudgmental service.

Prevention Point's early anarchistic, unfunded phase stretched from 1989 to 1991. Between 1991 and 1994, the organization sought and obtained funding from the city of San Francisco and at the same time was able to maintain a sense of autonomy and self-rule. Eventually, however, Prevention Point was forced to succumb to the demands and strictures of corporate non-profits, which directly conflicted with how Prevention Point had managed itself in its early years. Ironically, Prevention Point's greatest strength throughout its history—its anarchism and consensus approaches to decision making—proved to be a great weakness in the power struggles that developed with the non-profit organization that it established in order to have a legal supplier of syringes.

While Luis Kemnitzer was part of Prevention Point's first wave of involvement, Alex Kral is part of what he himself calls the "second wave." Kral, a public health epidemiologist and staff member at an AIDS research organization, arrived in San Francisco and became a Prevention Point volunteer in 1993. By that time, Prevention Point was already legitimate and officially protected by the mayor. Since 1991, the city had paid for Prevention Point's syringes and, through the San Francisco AIDS Foundation, it had provided a legally separate organization with part-time paid staff to assist the volunteers. Kral's memory of the events of the next two years tells the story of Prevention Point's attempt to maintain its original movement structure while conforming more and more to the demands of its funders. Kral's feelings about these developments is typical of many of Prevention Point's volunteer activists.

> The first wave of volunteers was basically a group of civil disobedient, anarchist people that kind of saw a need and just went ahead and did the work. And at that point, they met every week, I believe, as a group. And all decisions about the organization needed 100 percent consensus, and they didn't take any public funding. It was all privately funded in different ways. And I think they ran that way for a long time, until one day, as far as what I've heard anyway, George [Clark] became director, and I don't know exactly how, under what circumstances that was. But from what I hear from a lot of people, from a lot of the original people, one day George came to the meeting and had made the decision on his own . . . that he would take city funding. I think that was probably the biggest moment of change, because once you take public funding, then people ask you to do things differently. Then all of a sudden organizations need to be put into place, anarchy and consensus and all those things kind of get thrown out because funding agents want different things.[24]

According to Kral, from that moment on, some people stopped going to Prevention Point meetings in protest against taking city funding. However, they still considered the work of needle exchange important enough that they wanted to continue to do it. They said, "Well, I'm not going to have anything to do with this organization except for doing the work."[25] The decentralized nature of Prevention Point's work made it possible for activists to continue on as volunteers on the streets while distancing themselves from the organization as such.

By early 1993, Prevention Point had a budget, a paid director, and the other staff needed to organize supplies and coordinate volunteers. Officially, they were employees of a separate organization sheltered by SFAF called the HIV Prevention Project (HPP). Because the director, George Clark, had come from the Prevention Point ranks and was still an active volunteer, the differences between the grassroots movement and the formal organization were minimized. But to Kral and other newcomers, Prevention Point looked like a small non-profit:

> It was an organization like any other non-profit organization as far as I'm concerned. I saw no element of anarchy, I saw no element of, "We're doing something strange, or we're doing something not, you know, some civil disobedience" or any of that. I never had any sense of that. When I started I knew that it was, you know, semi-legal and I knew all that, but it really just, from when I started, I think it was an establishment.

In March 1994, Prevention Point decided to formalize the team meetings of the volunteers who actually did the distribution and exchange work to make sure that there was a regular check-in from every site every month. Each site selected someone to represent it, and the group as a whole was called the "participatory management team."

Some members of Prevention Point objected that creating this structure would establish a new "government" for the organization. The strongest supporters of the idea of participatory management were the "old timers" who felt that a formalized process would assure representation from all the spokes of the wheel. Two members of the team who were also volunteers (George and Yana) were involved in the reorganization. They supported the decision to allow members of the team to be paid $50 per meeting "voluntarily." (Some volunteers were opposed to the payment on the ground that it should be unnecessary.)

During the first year, the monthly meetings were used as a time for check-ins and updates, but no decisions of significance were made. Prevention Point's requirement that decisions be reached by consensus and its commitment to not making decisions for others kept these formal meetings from functioning in any sort of management mode overseeing the various sites. So long as the organization faced no crises, this lack of centralized management apparently worked well.

> I would bring up issues myself of things like distribution [giving out needles without requiring a one-for-one exchange]—some of the larger issues. Small issues are dealt with, you know. We've got a problem here; let's deal with it. But larger issues, like should we do a distribution rather than exchange, issues which were generally shot down by people as even discussion topics, you know. I wasn't even allowed to bring up that as a discussion topic. It was too much of an issue, or something.... But it really didn't change much as far as I'm concerned, after the PMT [participatory management team] started.[26]

In the fall of 1994, HPP hired a new executive director, the first who had not been a volunteer. This step marks the start of the third phase of Prevention Point's development: the movement's increasing subservience to a formal organization that had originally been created to serve it.

Roslyn Allen, the new director, came from Bayview Hunter's Point Foundation, an organization in a heavily African American area of San Francisco that originally had not approved of needle exchange, seeing it as a diversion from the more important goal of getting people off drugs altogether. She had never worked in a needle exchange program. Her primary substance-abuse experience was within a hierarchically organized non-profit serving the black community.

Alex Kral described the new director's style as top-down management. She rarely visited the exchange sites and only occasionally came to participatory management team meetings. To Prevention Point volunteers, the director's absence from participatory management team meetings was unacceptable. They compared her unfavorably to George Clark, who had been "one of us." After hearing other volunteers and members of the participatory management team complain about the situation for months, several decided to hold a meeting specifically to discuss the problem. As Alex Kral remembers,

> Well, the main reason I called the meeting was to have us figure out as the PMT, actually as Prevention Point, figure out what the role of PMT should be, what decision-making power it should have, and how it should go about getting that power. Because as it was I saw it as a kind of a pinball machine of people not really making decisions.
>
> Embedded in this whole concept or this whole meeting was that we had always thought, or it was always considered that the paid staff are working for Prevention Point in the sense that they are helping to make sure that Prevention Point runs the way it should. And they kind of help assist on a bigger [level], you know, whether it's office or getting the stuff . . . so that Prevention Point can do the work. That whole idea had flipped. So it seemed like we were all working for them, doing their work. We made a decision to exclude paid staff from the meeting because . . . the staff is HPP staff . . . . And there is a definite us and them.
>
> Rosalyn made her own [decision], without ever talking to any of us, to accept $100,000 from the city, through the AIDS Foundation, that the city demanded had to be spent on a women's site in the Mission and on a new site in the Western Addition. Now they came up with those ideas through the HIV Prevention Planning Committee . . . that made the decision to give Prevention Point money, never asking any of the volunteers, never asking any of the Prevention Point people what it is we need. Now it's pretty obvious that we're the people who would know best, I think, what would be necessary. And Rosalyn, very new in the job, just went to the meeting, and she said, "Okay, let's start a women's site in the Mission. Sure, we'll take the money." So she obviously is making the decisions . . . . [27]

Against this background and with the kind of resentment reflected in Kral's account of the events leading up to the meeting, thirteen people from among the seventy to eighty Prevention Point volunteers showed up, almost all of whom had other full-time jobs. The group agreed to prepare a letter summarizing their concerns and present it to the next participatory management team meeting, to which they would invite the director and the rest of the paid staff, now totaling four people. There was no formal consensus. When the letter was presented the following month, both the director and the rest of the paid staff expressed hurt and a sense of not being appreciated. According to Kral,

> Rosalyn ended up walking out of the meeting towards the end of it, and she said flat out, "If this is your process for getting these kinds of things, I'm not participating in it. I don't believe that you did this. I don't believe in this process. And this is going to make me want to change things less than more." That was her reaction, at which point the different people, PMT members who had been at that meeting, some of them started kind of back-pedaling and this and that, and it was kind of ugly. [28]

At this point the complaint process fizzled out. The Prevention Point volunteers, including those at the second meeting, did not want anything sent out without consensus, yet few had been at both meetings and many had been to none. Even those who had agreed to action at one time were unsure at a later time.

No letters were sent out, no formal action was taken by either Prevention Point, the HPP staff, or the two groups in unison. Informally, in the months following the confrontation, the director paid more attention to the Prevention Point volunteers, visiting sites more often and apparently listened to them more closely. But relative power relations were reaffirmed and not modified by the challenge. As for Kral,

> I've just decided that I'm not going to be part of the PMT process anymore myself, so I'm just quitting it all because I don't have the time to sit around anymore and not make decisions. And I felt I did a push to really make sure that some changes would happen in this organization, and it didn't really look like people were willing to do that. And so I'm bowing out of it altogether.

However, Kral decided to continue to work as a volunteer for Prevention Point and, in an anarchistic fashion, struggled to find additional resources for clients at his site. This continued to happen at the other sites as well.

> I've gotten a public health nurse now for our site, and I've got two new outreach workers with the city van, and we started giving out flu shots. And we're treating abscesses and providing all those kinds of [low-technology] medical services. Other sites have done different things. The Bayview site now is connected with a clinic and is able to give out some methadone maintenance detox slots for free. The women's site has childcare; Sixth Street has a doctor, med students and interns. All these things are site-specific. They're not, it's not through Prevention Point [or HPP], it's not through Prevention Point finding funding or finding these things or whatever. It's through the networks [of PP volunteers].

While he would prefer that the services were available or shared throughout the Prevention Point sites, Kral is resigned to not being heard.

> It seems to me that what Prevention Point has done from the beginning, and still is really only doing, the only thing that people really can all agree on is that there needs to be points [needles] gotten to people, that syringes need to get to people. I think that's it. I think that's really the only thing that everybody agrees on, and I don't think that there's anything else that people agree on. I think that at this point the only thing that Prevention Point is doing as a unity thing is getting out the syringes, the alcohol patch, e.g., supplies. That's all that it's doing. It's all it's ever been doing. As far as I'm concerned, what I want Prevention Point and the director to do is look into a whole host of other services and things to do for this population, because we've got a great base to reach a population that's not reachable in any other way. And they need a lot of different things.

My interview with Alex Kral took place in November of 1995, when Prevention Point was stuck at the stage of organizational development in which the "work groups" (site volunteers) were comfortable with one another in a horizontal network but were unable to effectively utilize the non-profit structure which was designed to help them with funding. Anarchism and consensus management have worked well for Prevention Point if one thinks primarily of the numbers of needles exchanged; but to utilize their new financial resources, the volunteers might need a system of linkages and influence that would better connect them in fact, with power, to the world of non-profit funding.

....

Foucault in the Streets:
New York City
Act(s) UP

In 1988, I attended ACT-UP meetings in New York City for three months. ACT-UP (AIDS Coalition To Unleash Power) represents a direct-action response to the epidemic reminiscent of the Student Non-Violent Coordinating Committee (SNCC), Students for a Democratic Society (SDS), and some elements of gay liberation and the women's movement. The similarity is not too surprising since many of the founders and early activists of ACT-UP cut their political teeth on these movements. In some ways, ACT-UP is a response to the bureaucratization and mainstreaming of earlier AIDS activism.[1]

What is most striking about ACT-UP to many people is its effective use of graphics and media, an "in your face" style of direct action and, at the same time, an ability to negotiate with leaders in government and the health field using sophisticated technical analysis.[1a] The New York City organization combined these diverse strategies successfully due to its class and race base, its initial location in New York, and the movement pasts of its leaders.

Many male and female ACT-UP members describe themselves as radical in interviews and in their own writing. Older members often state that their identity and their commitments to direct action were forged in either the civil rights movement of the sixties or the gay movement of the seventies. The connections to civil rights and the feminist movement were cited by several women that I interviewed in 1989. The men referred more often to the New York gay movement of the seventies. A number of New York ACT-UP's senior leaders were also members of the Gay Activists Alliance, formed in 1969 and committed to a gay-focused movement. Many men also acknowledge the powerful influence of the civil rights movement. ACT-UP organizational practice is ultra-democratic, modeled on the anti-nuclear movement of the seventies, with a meeting structure designed to allow all to participate and to keep the process moving.

ACT-UP, as an organization with a predominantly well-educated, white, and gay leadership, has also been affected both directly and indirectly by the new "queery theory." This theory is itself heavily dependent on the work of French critical and "post-modern" theorists, especially Michel Foucault, who wrote extensively on sexuality, representation, and the maintenance of social control through public rules of discourse. Foucault's radical analysis, as well as his identity as a gay man, has made him and his work objects of sustained attention by gay intellectuals and activists. His theoretical sophistication and attention to the body as a site of political struggle mirror the practice of New York City ACT-UP.[2]

ACT-UP's explicit politics are not based on identity ("being gay," "having AIDS"), but its New York members were overwhelmingly drawn from a distinct cultural base which had been developed through identity politics. The cultural base was that of the well-educated, white, gay male of Manhattan who had sophisticated knowledge of New York's culture, politics, and art. In this chapter we see that the functional consequence of combining radical intent with a cultural base whose class and race privilage are not examined is to reassert and privilege the concerns and aesthetics of whites and men. ACT-UP was able to step outside a limited political discourse on AIDS in order to present its radical approach, but it remained trapped in a liberal perspective on the involvement of women, the poor, and people of color in its own movement and organization.[2a]

The Beginnings

In terms of its proximate causes, we can understand the founding of ACT-UP as a response to frustrations with the Gay Men's Health Crisis (GMHC), New York City's premier AIDS education and service non-profit organization. GMHC was founded in 1982 by Larry Kramer, Paul Popham, and others. According to Kramer, he handled the daily management of the organization.[3] In his book, *Reports from the Holocaust: The Making of an AIDS Activist*, Kramer sets the stage for the birth of ACT-UP by discussing changes at the Gay Men's Health Crisis. From the start, Kramer admits, he was "out to attack every perceived enemy in sight."[4] Initially, Kramer thought GMHC would be a political response to the epidemic as well as a temporary provider of services. He became increasingly frustrated as his dreams and hopes were repeatedly dashed. As early as 1983, in "1,112 and Counting," published in the *New York Native*, Kramer raised all the difficult issues that continue to make AIDS a crisis today: its concentration among disenfranchised groups, waiting lists at hospitals, the bureaucracy of the Centers for Disease Control,[5] always a "new" set of treatments, and the need for access. Prefiguring his later writing, Kramer drew an analogy between the AIDS epidemic and the Holocaust:

> I am sick of "men" who say, "We've got to keep quiet or *they* will do such and such."
> *They* usually means the straight majority, the "Moral" Majority, or similarly perceived representatives of *them*. Okay, you "men"—be my guests: You can march off now to the gas chambers; just get right in line.
> We shall always have enemies. Nothing we can ever do will remove them. Southern newspapers and Jerry Falwell's publications are already printing editorials proclaiming AIDS as God's deserved punishment on homosexuals. So what: Nasty words make poor little sissy pansy wilt and die?

By the time Kramer compiled *Reports from the Holocaust,* he felt that although many of the founders of GMHC were motivated by essentially political concerns and community survival, this was not true of those who followed. Many, he argued, "were not 'activists' at all; they were concerned citizens who wished to help quietly, in the pastoral sense.[5a] And so continued the concretizing of GMHC into its present state: that of a social service organization, rather than an advocacy one."

By 1987, Kramer was one of the most verbal critics of GMHC, publicly pleading with the organization to become more politically active and less of a service organization. In an open letter to GMHC, published in the *Native,* Kramer poured out his frustration.

I cannot for the life of me understand how the organization I helped form has become such a bastion of conservatism and such a bureaucratic mess. The bigger you get, the more cowardly you become; the more money you receive, the more self-satisfied you are.

Most of GMHC's efforts are devoted to providing services the city should be providing and would probably be forced to provide if GMHC were not in existence. This is not to say you are not providing them better than the city would; you are. But in taking our money, you are, in essence, asking us to pay twice for what you are doing—once in our contributions to you, and once in our taxes to this city. Thus you should be providing for us additional services our city will never provide—gay service, gay leadership. You don't. You have become simply another city social service agency, and at the rate one hears about your inner squabblings, the rapidly declining quality of the staff you are hiring, and the increasing unhappiness of those who work for you, it will not be long before you are indistinguishable from any of the city departments—Health, Police, Parking Violations—that serve our city so tepidly . . . .

Our only salvation lies in aggressive scientific research. This will come only from political pressure. Every dime for research that we've had has come only from hard political fighting.

Thus all our solutions can only be achieved through political action. All the kindness in the world will not stem this epidemic. Only political action can change the course of events.[6]

Others in New York were clearly in agreement. Five years into the epidemic, community organizations had grown, but government and medical solutions had not provided the magic cure so eagerly sought. In addition, drugs with some potential seemed tantalizingly close, but their availability was limited and too expensive.

In March 1987, these conditions and a specific set of events led to the founding of ACT-UP, an organization eager for HIV/AIDS political action. In 1989 Vito Russo, then active in ACT-UP, recalled:

When I came home to New York from San Francisco I discovered that there was a sort of battle beginning over the role of the Gay Men's Health Crisis, which was the only organization, and it was mostly instigated by Larry Kramer, who was saying that he had been one of the founders of the Gay Men's Health Crisis with the idea in mind that it would be an overtly political organization. And it didn't work out that way. It became immediately a social service agency which did all the things that the city, state, and federal government was not doing or funding. And there was a definite need for that. But there was no confrontational role. There was no street activist role. There was no civil disobedience role. There was no direct action role. And so Larry Kramer called a town meeting at the community center to say essentially, "What we need in this city is a group of committed activists who are willing to do direct action around issues of AIDS." And that's how ACT-UP was born and began to meet every week.[7]

During that speech Kramer told the audience that he had just found out about new drugs whose availability was being delayed because of red tape. He criticized GMHC for its inadequate response to this situation and went on to propose what became the key to the emergence of the new organization: "We need to do something and not just criticize them. We need to each begin to act, to pick up the pieces of paper that collectively make trash in the streets." In response to this urging, those in the audience decided to have an action meeting two days later. Consistent reports state that 300 people showed up at the Lesbian and Gay Community Center and founded ACT-UP.

While ACT-UP quickly became a national organization, the major organizational ancestors of ACT-UP were all in New York City, the long-time home of most of its founders. Of these, the single most important organization was the Gay Activists Alliance (GAA). As Vito Russo recalled in 1989, GAA from its start was involved in direct action and media activism.

Almost virtually all our demonstrations were in reaction to some homophobic thing that had happened, and we needed to go after them—so that, for instance, a man named Joseph Epstein wrote a piece in *Harper's* magazine about homosexuality, and he said things like, "If I had the power I would wish homosexuality off the face of the earth." And we picked up on that, and we decided that we would have a major zap against *Harper's*. And our goals were to get an article written by an openly gay person sort of countering Joseph Epstein and to get the magazine to stop publishing homophobic pieces. And so a big demonstration was planned around that, and we took over the offices of *Harper's* magazine. And that was one of our most successful actions.

And then we found out, for instance, that there was an organization in New York called Fidelifax, and what they did was illegal. They would, for $12.50, believe it or not, investigate the private life of an employee for a prospective employer, to see if there was any dirt about them, like if they were gay, you know, or something like that. And we knew that according to the New York State Charter this was not legal. So I mean to us it was clearly illegal that there should be an organization in business which investigated the private lives of people for their employers.

And so what we did was we called them up and we said, "You investigate people and you reveal that they're homosexual to prospective employers," and they said, "Yes." And we said, "Well, how do you know if a person's gay? What kind of research do you do?" And the guy said, "Well, if it walks like a duck and talks like a duck and acts like a duck it must be a duck."

And so we dressed up Marty Robinson in a duck costume and we went down there and we picketed them, and Bela Abzug at the time joined us. And she said, "I've checked the law on this." She's a lawyer, and she said, "This is illegal. They can't do this." And we had the New York State Commission revoke their license and put them out of business.[8]

According to Russo, the GAA invented the political use of the term "zap." When I asked him what it meant exactly, he replied,

To zap someone . . . is to corner him in a public place and to, you know, ask redress for grievances. A zap is an action. I mean ACT-UP calls them actions, you know, "We're going to discuss actions now." And sometimes on the floor people will get up and say, "We have this action we want to do, and this is who we're going to zap."[9]

ACT-UP shared other important features with GAA, most strikingly its single issue focus. GAA itself was an outgrowth of the Gay Liberation Front (GLF), a radical organization of men and women formed in New York City shortly after the 1969 Stonewall uprising. GAA's members, including Russo, left the GLF in 1969 over debates concerning GLF support for the Black Panthers, who were openly homophobic.

In his closely researched account of GLF, Terence Kissack notes the single focus of the GAA and some of the crucial differences between these two seminal organizations, differences that presaged contemporary debate among AIDS activists about focus and diversity. Kissack writes,

To assure that the Alliance would not become embroiled in movement politics, the group's constitution carried a bylaw that stated the alliance "will not endorse, ally with, or otherwise support any political party, candidate for public office, and/or any organization not directly related to the homosexual cause." The alliance had elected officers and clear rules for membership and expulsion. Its meetings were run according to Robert's Rules of Order. To those who stayed in the Gay Liberation Front, the Gay Activists Alliance's politics were antidemocratic, hierarchical, and inequitable and served to reinforce the power relations that they were trying to overthrow . . . . While the Gay Activists Alliance attacked misrepresentation of homosexuality in mainstream media, Front members focused much of their efforts on the alternative press.[10]

The GAA, which had an extensive cultural program and fewer intense conflicts, because its enemies were more easily distinguished, grew and became the model of gay organizations in New York and elsewhere, while the GLF was essentially moribund in two years. Almost all of the older gay activists of ACT-UP with gay political pasts traced their roots to GAA.

Kramer saw the purpose of ACT-UP as "originally . . . fighting for the release of experimental drugs. (I say 'originally' because its interests have now broadened to include other items and I feel they've lost a bit of focus on the drug issue, which for me is just about the main issue of paramount importance.)"[11]

This is also Vito Russo's recollection:

> . . . Basically our goal in ACT-UP was to get experimental drugs and treatments and substances which looked promising but were not toxic into the bodies of sick people as quickly as possible. Our goal was to move the FDA [Food and Drug Administration] forward, to move the NIH [National Institutes of Health) forward, and to stop the AIDS crisis by any means—that's in our charter, what we wrote when we got together. And we would stop at nothing and that we would be willing to be arrested; we would be willing to commit civil disobedience; we would be willing to break the law in order to achieve our goals and attract media attention to this issue.[12]

In later intraorganizational conflicts, one side was often represented as those whose primary concern was "getting drugs into bodies" and the other side as those who had other interests as well.

On March 24, 1987, ACT-UP held its first demonstration, or to use its own language, its first "action." Several hundred people demonstrated on Wall Street against the Food and Drug Administration and Burroughs Wellcome, the pharmaceutical company that manufactured AZT. The FDA had given the company a monopoly on sales of AZT and allowed the corporation to charge patients more than $10,000 annually for the medication. At the time, AZT was believed to be the only treatment that could slow the replication of HIV and delay death from AIDS.[13] In his 1989 account, Kramer indicates the role of the media in making the demonstration work and in bringing ACT-UP into national prominence almost instantly.

> Joseph Papp (head of the New York Public Theater) contributed an effigy (built in his workshops) of Dr. Frank Young, the head of the FDA, who was "hung" in front of Trinity Church. Some 250 men and women tied up traffic for several hours and passed out tens of thousands of fact sheets about the FDA horror show, as well as copies of my *Times* op-ed piece . . . [criticizing the FDA, Burroughs Wellcome, and NIH]. The demonstration and subsequent arrests made the national nightly newscasts, and when, several weeks later, Dr. Young made some promises (which he has yet to keep) about speedier drug testing and release, Dan Rather gave credit to ACT-UP. It was a wonderful beginning.[14]

On April 15, only three weeks later, ACT-UP held its second demonstration at the New York main post office, where hundreds were waiting in line to file their tax returns. It was at this demonstration that the famous slogan "Silence = Death" first appeared.

During the next seven months, New York ACT-UP held nine major demonstrations, was cloned in several cities, and produced a variety of graphics. The organization developed its signature style quickly—both organizationally and externally.

The speed and efficiency with which ACT-UP became effective was made possible by the increasing degree of organization within the gay community of New York and, for that matter, nationally. This social complexity was in turn the result of the gay liberation movement of the seventies and the proliferation of AIDS organizations that were predominantly gay or at least open about and supportive of gay people, especially gay men. The melding of gay institutions with AIDS organizations had set the social context for the founding of ACT-UP. The leaders of most AIDS organizations at this time were gay men, as were the great majority of AIDS cases, over 80 percent in New York City. Additionally most of the people identified in the United States as having AIDS were also white. ACT-UP began as a predominantly gay, white, male organization with politically experienced leaders.

Process and Activism

One of the major strengths of ACT-UP has been its ability to provide a home for people with very diverse politics and commitments of time. This has been accomplished through a flexible structure and decision-making process.

The core of the organization and its decision making is in the Monday night meeting (replicated in almost every ACT-UP-type group). These gatherings, based on the mass meeting model, developed a structure and process designed to keep the meeting moving, provide interesting moments, build solidarity, and foster participation in both future meetings and public actions. By the fall of 1989, the pattern was well established.

New York City meetings were held in the main meeting room of the Lesbian and Gay Community Center in Chelsea, the heart of the organized white gay community. Entering the room, one passed tables of materials, especially xeroxes of newspaper articles and letters to newspapers by ACT-UP members, flyers and information sheets for upcoming or recent zaps and actions, announcements of other organizations' AIDS-related events, stickers, the ACT-UP weekly calendar and contact sheet, *The Weekly Report* of ACT-UP, and posters. In short, enough paper per person to raise environmental concerns, but deeply satisfying to an information junkie such as myself. All materials on the tables were free.

The meeting began with a weekly ritual in which the co-facilitators (one male and one female) led the audience in a recital of the ACT-UP statement of purpose:

> ACT-UP is a diverse, non-partisan group united in anger and committed to direct action to end the AIDS crisis. We protest and demonstrate; we meet with government and public health officials; we research and distribute the latest medical information; **we are not silent.**

Applause followed. Activists asked members of the police to identify themselves. (None ever did.) The meeting proceeded, following Robert's Rules of Order. The group welcomed new members; everyone present for the first time was asked to stand. New members were applauded by the group, and individuals assigned responsibility for new members passed them membership sheets to sign. These opening rituals reaffirmed the community aspect of the organization, required identification of new attendees, began their incorporation, and brought a group focus and participation into the room.

All meetings followed a standardized schedule, with normally effective attempts to keep within a two-hour time frame, even for the most important matters. Announcements were organized into groups of five, and announcers went to the front of the room to speed things up and to make themselves visible as well. Committee reports were next. At the time I attended meetings, there were ten major committees as well as various ad hoc groups and caucuses. Not every committee had something to report each week.

Next came proposals for zaps and actions. In ACT-UP language, zaps are actions that can be organized within a week. An action is a more elaborate zap and may involve extensive media and other organizing work requiring several months to plan and execute. After all the proposals had been heard and voted on, those wishing to work on them left the main room to make a plan. In this way, ACT-UP members literally voted with their feet to determine the amount of resources to be given to any particular project.

Although actions had to be approved by consensus at the Monday night meetings, those which were rejected could be pursued by an affinity group. Vito Russo describes the affinity group process and how it resulted in the invention of the "Silence = Death" T-shirt.

> There's always issues that come to the floor that need a vote—the general membership votes on everything. Committees decide what they want to do . . . . For instance the action committee is the hottest committee, because it plans all our actions. And they'll go away and people who are willing to go to committee meetings will decide what they'd like to do next. And then they have to bring it to the floor on Monday night and it has to be a floor vote, so that there's consensus. And if anything gets voted down by the floor that maybe ten or twelve people still feel very strongly about and still want to do, they form what's called an *affinity group*. And that means that these people, acting as a group but not as part of ACT-UP, are going to go ahead and do this, whether anybody likes it or not.
>
> And so detractors of ACT-UP . . . are always saying, "You know, this business of affinity groups. You might say that they're not ACT-UP, but they're ACT-UP. And every time the floor votes something down, a dozen people go off and do it anyway." And the point, according to me of course, is that they do it very well. And usually, not always, but usually when an affinity group goes off and does something on its own, they come back to the organization and they are applauded by the organization for what they've done.
>
> I mean, for instance, an affinity group made up the logo "Silence = Death" and made the T-shirts and chose the colors and designed it. They are a graphics committee. And they didn't do this with the approval of the membership; they came one night to a Monday night meeting, with these shirts and they said, "We made this up, and we want to know what you think of it," and everybody went, "Oh, it's fabulous. These are great." And it became the logo of the organization. But they didn't have permission from the floor because there were objections from the floor. "Oh, yeah, right. Now we're going to start selling T-shirts. What else would you like to do—you want to make cof-

fee cups with our logo on it?" So this was like a huge thing that got voted down. These people went off and did it anyway, and it turned out to be a success.[15]

Sometimes, however, when a proposed action was defeated in the general meeting, it stayed defeated. Russo again:

> Last Christmas we had an idea that we wanted to go to the Macy's ... Thanksgiving Day Parade, and that at a certain point along the route, just before Macy's, that we would have our own float hidden on 38th Street, and that we would drive it into the parade. And that it would be a float of Silence = Death, and that of course they would stop us and they would arrest us, but not before we got on TV, because the television cameras are on Herald Square ....
>
> And then people started saying things like, you know, first of all Santa Claus is the last float in the Thanksgiving Day Parade, because that's the opening of the Christmas season. And people were saying they were going to pour blood on Santa Claus [laughter]. Then people started saying, "Wait a minute. I want to know what Thanksgiving Day Parade has to do with AIDS. And why are we choosing this forum." And I said, "Because everybody's going to be watching the Thanksgiving Day Parade on TV. It's the perfect opportunity. They won't be able to miss this." And they're saying, "This is ridiculous. There are thousands of children out there. You're going to pour blood on Santa Claus. [Laughter.] This is the wrong forum for this kind of expression." And, in fact, ultimately it never got done. (A) Because the floor voted it down, and (B) because there was no affinity group powerful enough to organize something on such a mass level.[16]

The distinctive nature of ACT-UP's public actions arose from its combination of direct action, civil disobedience, a focus on mainstream media, and its striking use of graphics. This combination was blended together like gunpowder and a charge, which was shot at targets that were determined to be obstructing a rapid response to the epidemic. The other side of ACT-UP's activism was less visible but was equally important: its role within the scientific and medical establishment.

ACT-UP's impact has ranged from changes in public policy at the local level in many cities and countries around the world to its successful re-orientation of the federal drug approval process and the incorporation of drug consumers on NIH and FDA review panels. ACT-UP's success has been due in no small way to its race, gender, and class composition, i.e., because it has so many highly educated white male members. Just as their artistic knowledge, skill, and contacts were effective in using the media, so also was their education and class composition effective in working the medical side of the street. As a predominantly middle- and upper-middle-class, gay, white, and desperate group with a decade of gay culture, politics, and institutions to support it, ACT-UP was able to bring a wide variety of resources to bear on the institutions it identified as obstacles to its goals.[16a]

ACT-UP also appealed to younger gay men and lesbians drawn to activist expression of their identity, even when the epidemic itself was not as much of a life focus as it was for the generation of gay men in their thirties and forties. By 1992 there were over 100 documented ACT-UP chapters in the U.S. and internationally.[17]

In its first year alone ACT-UP organized or participated in the following demonstrations:[18]

June 1	Third International Conference on AIDS, Washington D.C.: Police wearing bright yellow rubber gloves arrest sixty-four protesters from various activist groups. Key issues addressed in handouts: national education campaign; legislation to prohibit discrimination in employment, housing, insurance and health care.[19] Graphics: AIDSGATE graphic produced ("54% of PWAs are black or Hispanic. AIDS #1 killer of women between ages of 24-29 in NYC. Genocide of all non-whites, non-males, and non-heterosexuals?") (DemoGraphics: 34, 36).
June 28	New York annual gay pride parade. ACT-UP float represents AIDS "quarantine camp."[20]
June 30	Demonstration at Federal Plaza in New York City. Over thirty people arrested. Key issues addressed in handouts: Social Security benefits denied to PWAs; nation/state-wide mandatory testing bills.[21]
July 21-24	Around-the-clock vigil at Memorial Sloan-Kettering Hospital, a federally designated AIDS Treatment and Ed-ucation Unit (ATEU).
July 26	Demonstration at St. Patrick's Cathedral, in response to Reagan's naming of Cardinal John O'Connor to the Presidential Commission on HIV Epidemic (PCHE).[22]
August 4	Action at Northwest Airline's New York office: To protest the airline's refusal to allow passage to PWAs.[23]
September 9	ACT-UP demonstration in Washington.[24]
October	March on Washington for Lesbian and Gay Rights: ACT NOW (AIDS Coalition to Network, Organize and Win) in Washington D.C. formed.
December 10	Affinity group that calls itself "Metropolitan Health Association" makes appointment with Health Commissioner Joseph, then occupies his office. Eight arrested.[25]

1988

January	Women's Committee forms within ACT-UP, in response to *Cosmopolitan* article.[26]
January 19	*Cosmo* demonstration at Hearst Magazine building. Nearly 150 people shouting, handing out condoms and fliers, call for boycott of magazine. *Graphics: "AIDS: 1 in 61" poster by Gran Fury, in English and Spanish. Key issues: racism and AIDS.[27]

*Beginning of production of documentary, "Doctors, Liars, and Women: AIDS Activists Say No to *Cosmo*" by ACT-UP Women's Committee.

February 15   Demonstration at Presidential Commission on the HIV epidemic hearings, New York. Graphics: "He Kills Me" poster (attacking President Reagan) appears.[28]

Spring   "Let the Record Show" installation in New Museum of Contemporary Art concerning AIDS. Afterwards, Gran Fury forms as a committee within ACT-UP.[29]

March 24   Wall Street II. 111 arrested. Key issues: Drug research and availability; federal funds spent on AIDS education; legislative attacks on PWAs; lack of presidential attention. Graphics: Gran Fury's money/bills graphics appear, as does "AID$ NOW" poster.[30]

April 29-May 7   "Spring AIDS Action." ACT NOW affinity group coordinates actions which last nine days in New York, Albany, and Newark, NJ. Key issues: Homophobia, PWAs, people of color, substance abuse, prisons, women, worldwide crisis, testing and treatment. ACT-UP proposes national day of protest at state legislatures. Graphics: Gran Fury produces All People With AIDS Are Innocent.[31]

April 29   Kiss-In—public demonstration and celebration of gay and lesbian sexuality: GRAPHICS: Gran Fury's "Read My Lips" posters, the lesbian side is challenged by ACT-UP women, and then changed on the T-shirt images.[32]

April 30   Action at University Hospital in Newark over its neglect of the needs of PWAs. ACT-UP demands that the hospital commence clinical trials of experimental drugs, provide HIV patients with list of clinical trial sites, and that the state allocate research funds.

May 1   Action to reach out to black and Hispanic churches. Letters to pastors.

May 2	Action with ADAPT to focus on substance abuse. Rally at City Hall. Issues: free needles; expansion of drug treatment and outreach prevention programs; housing.
May 3	Action at Harlem State Office Building, State Office of Corrections. Issues: segregation of incarcerated PWAs; poor health care; lack of education and condoms and needles; forced HIV testing. Graphics: AIDS BEHIND BARS by Gran Fury.
May 4	Action around women's issues, organized by Women's Committee, focus on sexual transmission. Visits to New York high schools, street education outside the schools. Graphics: SEXISM REARS ITS UNPROTECTED HEAD poster by Gran Fury (criticized by NYC ACT-UP women as too phallic.) In the evening, an action at a Mets game, with information, condoms, and unfurled banners in three different sections of the stadium seating: STRIKE OUT AIDS; NO GLOVE NO LOVE; DON'T BALK AT SAFER SEX. MEN, USE CONDOMS OR BEAT IT graphics designed, but not used at demos (DemoGraphics: 62-65).
May 5	Action at International Bldg. at Rockefeller Center, to call attention to international AIDS crisis. Issues: U.S. world leadership; WHO past dues; increased U.S. funding to WHO; increased U.S. aid to Africa; ceasing of mandatory HIV testing; comprehensive AIDS policy.
May 6	Action at FAO Schwartz, focus on testing and treatment issues. Issues: first federally funded clinic for pediatric AIDS, in which half babies receive placebos.
May 7	Action in Albany, display of New York Names Project quilt. Vito Russo speech targets state inaction. Issues: hate crime legislation (lesbian and gay men); affordable housing, adequate support services, skilled nursing facilities for PWAs; education; increased funding for drug rehabilitation and clean needle education; prisoners' rights.[33]

A key factor in ACT-UP's success has been its ability to move back and forth between the streets, the galleries and other cultural institutions, and the media, all of which was due to its members' gay connections and penetration into the cultural and media worlds of New York. For example, ACT-UP's art show at the New Museum of Contemporary Art in New York was arranged by Bill Olander, a curator there and a member of ACT-UP.[34] As for the famous ACT-UP graphics, the originals were made by a group that included well-established commercial and fine artists. This level of access to the arts and culture in a city that prided itself on being the center of art and culture, together with a strong taste for the streets, led to a highly effective blending of representation and action in ACT-UP, both in fact and theory. The group of graphic and fine artists who came together as the Gran Fury Collective was formed directly out of ACT-UP, according to Richard Meyer, and was

> devoted to the ongoing production of AIDS activist imagery . . . . They took the name Gran Fury, a reference both to their own rage in the midst of the epidemic and, somewhat campily, to the specific model of the Plymouth sedan that the New York City Police use as squad cars. Although several commercial and fine artists were part of the collective, so too were a hairdresser, a costume designer, an architect, a filmmaker, and a nurse.[35]

During its life and work with ACT-UP, the Gran Fury Collective created the ACT-UP dollars used in the Wall Street demonstrations of 1988, the "Read My Lips" posters, the widely-distributed "Kissing Doesn't Kill" bus posters, "Sexism Rears Its Unprotected Head," "Use Condoms or Beat It," "The Government Has Blood on Its Hands," and the fake *New York Times* paper ["New York Crimes"] which ACT-UP wrapped around the real *New York Times* and slipped into newspaper stands.

In addition to its Gran Fury Collective and other internal artists, again according to Meyer, ACT-UP was able to draw on support from a wide variety of people and institutions, including the contemporary artists David Hockney and Keith Haring and the Museum of Contemporary Art. Though it was an unincorporated organization that regularly broke the law via civil disobedience, ACT-UP raised enormous sums of money. During 1988, ACT-UP New York raised $300,000 and, in the following year, $600,000.[36]

ACT-UP focused its organizing strictly on AIDS the same way that GAA focused its work on homophobia and the development of a pro-gay culture. ACT-UP members saw not "just" an epidemic, but an epidemic that was hard to stop because of political and social bigotry. Vito Russo comments:

> Ray Navarro [psychologist and New York AIDS activist] said something in Philadelphia this week that I thought was really interesting and good to say, and profound. And that's that the reason why we have an AIDS crisis and not an AIDS epidemic is homophobia, racism, and sexism. If those three issues didn't exist, we would be dealing with an epidemic. But because of homophobia, racism, and sexism, we're dealing with a crisis. And so those are going to determine, more than almost anything else, the future of ACT-UP as a group. The nature of the epidemic in terms of minority communities and government inaction and unresponsiveness . . .[37]

Despite its sophisticated understanding of the politics of the epidemic and good intentions to reach out beyond the gay community, ACT-UP's leadership was itself limited. Though these activists would readily feel comfortable with calling themselves gay and male, few would think of adding "white" to their self-description. The lack of consciousness about race reflects a common pattern. To dominant groups, their dominance is so "natural," so self-evident, that they take over the category, for example, the category "gay," without noticing the exclusion of others (for example, non-white men). The cultural composition of the white Gran Fury Collective had a dramatic effect on ACT-UP's materials and its efforts to reach out to women and communities of color.

When one examines ACT-UP graphics, zaps, actions, and rhetoric, the salience of discourse on race, sexism, and sexuality becomes clear. Despite its flexible structure and process, and despite its goals, ACT-UP, like many movement organizations, had internal problems with sexism and racism. Ironically, in addition, the presumably democratic decision-making processes and a biased system of access to resources fostered maintenance of racial domination by giving a greater weight to white, male, and gay values in the graphic representations of the organization. This is ironic since it was clearly *not* the intent of ACT-UP to support white or male hegemony.

ACT-UP's "democratic" way of determining resource allocation (i.e., vote with your feet) ensured that most resources would flow to projects that reflected the values and concerns of the majority. Most of the famous AIDS images were developed by predominantly white, male work groups to accompany actions approved by consensus of the entire organization. Many of the best graphics represent a predominantly gay, white, and male approach to the issue presented. It should be remembered, and not as a criticism, that this organization, while focused on a wider epidemic affecting straight people as well as gay men and lesbians, was essentially a gay organization, formed at the gay community center and meeting there regularly. It is reasonable for the organization to especially examine and respond to the aspects of AIDS that affected its members in terms of their own vulnerabilities—one of which is their stigmatized identity—and their strengths, which here include education, media sophistication, and access to money.

An examination of some of the most famous ACT-UP posters demonstrates the ways that this prioritization was expressed in the organization's graphics. In its early poster containing the most famous ACT-UP image, "Silence = Death," created and first displayed in 1987, the small print, which criticizes the CDC, the FDA, and the Vatican, reads:

> Why is Reagan silent about AIDS? What is really going on at the Centers for Disease Control, the Federal Drug Administration, and the Vatican? Gays and lesbians are not expendable .... Use your power .... Vote .... Boycott .... Defend yourselves .... Turn anger, fear, grief, into action.[38]

The only cultural groups affected by AIDS deemed worth mentioning are gays and lesbians. Everyone else, presumably, is expendable. [Illustration 6.1]

Bright bold graphics are typical of the materials generated by ACT-UP and Gran Fury, its graphics affinity group, as in the bull's-eye image of "He Kills Me," the Ronald Reagan poster carried on a picket line in February 1988, protesting the Presidential Commission Hearing in New York City. [Illustration 6.2] The 1989 campaign against the politics of New York's Catholic Church and Cardinal

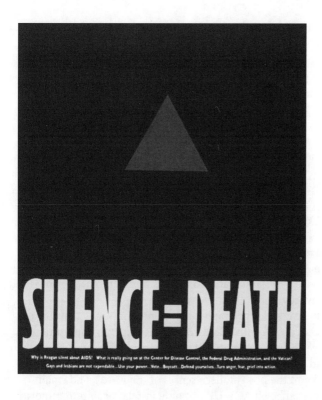

Illustration 6.1:
Silence = Death (Silence = Death Project, 1987). Colors are bright pink triangle on black background with white lettering.

Illustration 6.2: *He Kills Me (Donald Moffett, 1987). Colors are orange and black bullseye, with orange lettering.*

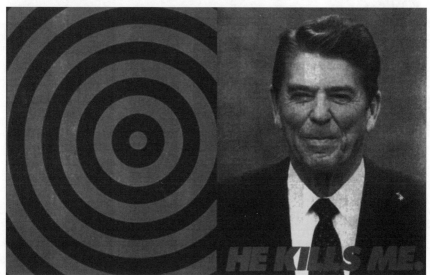

O'Connor was marked by direct action, bright graphics, and humor. Under the condom, in the "Know Your Scumbag" poster, the text reads "This one prevents AIDS," a reference to the Cardinal's influence in preventing sex education and condom distribution in public schools. [Illustration 6.3]

In these examples, the "neutral," unmarked category of a person with AIDS most often represented the interests, sensibilities, and priorities of middle-class white gay men and only secondarily the interests of people of color, women, or the poor.

The materials generated by the organization during the same period (1986-1990), as part of campaigns to address the needs of the poor, of women, and people of color, present a different esthetic—in many cases much less eye-catching or pleasing. Images 6:4 to 6:7 are posters designed for these more marginalized populations. In the poster "We Die—They Do Nothing!" only a close reading tells the viewer that this poster is about people of color. [Illustration 6.4] It was printed in black and white on cheap paper. The poster, "AIDS: 1 in 61," is one of the few bilingual graphics from ACT-UP. The theme is the heterosexual epidemic and the children born infected—1 in 61. [Illustration 6.5] This poster, too, was printed in black and white and is wordy.

What these very different styles of graphic representation say is that life as a gay white man is energetic, confrontive, and zippy. It is colorful, and humorous and filled with the power of resistance. But life as a person of color is presented as depressing, black and white (and maybe a little red), wordy, dull, hard to read (in both the traditional and the post-modern senses of the word), and small.

Representational issues affected ACT-UP not only in relationship to minority and poor populations, but also in terms of women. A conflict and revision of a Gran Fury poster designed for the women's focus day of the Nine Days of Action in Spring, 1988, signals both the complications of and solutions to sexism within ACT-UP.

Gran Fury unanimously approved "Sexism Rears Its Unprotected Head," which Richard Meyer describes as a "monumentally erect penis surrounded by three slogans" for use for women's day. The poster was "received with marked ambivalence by some members of ACT-UP, especially by several women who felt the graphic glorified phallic power more forcefully than it encouraged safer sex." [Illustration 6.6] Gran Fury then made a crack and peel sticker to replace it, using one of the slogans, "Men Use Condoms or Beat It," which punned visually on the yellow traffic signs "Men at Work," as well as on the double meanings of "beat it." [Illustration 6.7]

This male dominance should not be taken to imply that the women of ACT-UP were passive reactors. Instead they were involved in leadership, zaps, and actions of all sorts. At various times the weekly meetings were co-chaired by women; there was a women's issues committee and also a women's caucus. The women made videos, wrote flyers, organized demonstrations, and worked effectively to bring ACT-UP members to demonstrations with other organizations

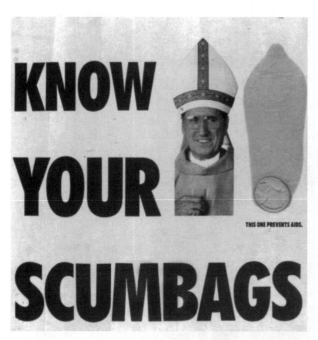

Illustration 6.3: Know Your Scumbags (Richard Deagle and Victor Mendolia, 1989). Colors: bright red lettering, pink condom, red, white, and black photo.

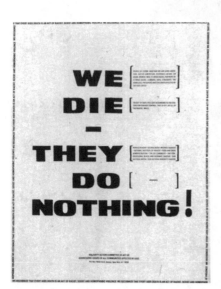

Illustration 6.4: We Die—They Do Nothing! (Gran Fury, 1988). Colors are black and white.

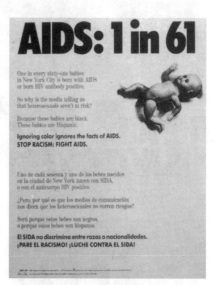

Illustration 6.5: AIDS: 1 in 61 (Gran Fury, 1988). Colors are black and white.

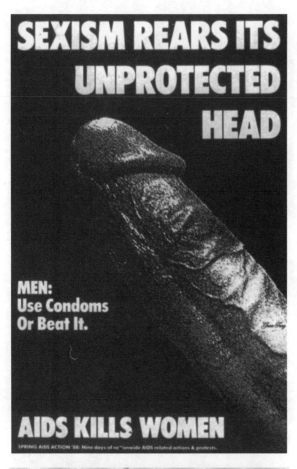

Illustration 6.6: Sexism Rears its Unprotected Head (Gran Fury, 1988). Colors are black and white.

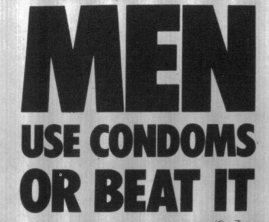

Illustration 6.7: Men Use Condoms or Beat it (Gran Fury, 1988). Colors are yellow background and black lettering.

that addressed women's issues. They were the prime movers in the successful national policy activism to expand the list of AIDS-defining conditions to include illnesses such as recurrent vaginitis and cervical cancer that specifically affect women, and they led the struggle to gain access for women to drug trials. Their book, *Women, AIDS, & Activism*, documents their work and philosophy.[39]

The differences between the "white male" posters and the others is in the materials and colors used and the originality and effectiveness of the graphic design. This is not a matter of esthetics or ethnic or gender difference per se, but of access to materials and technical resources. Most ACT-UP posters were developed by predominantly gay white male groups, with input only by way of reaction and revision from women and people of color. The materials produced are also stronger when they focus on male, gay, and white issues.

But why should this prioritization matter as we look at the graphic legacy of ACT-UP? Primarily because an organization claiming to speak only—and especially—about the most basic AIDS issues produced its best work for one segment of the population affected by the epidemic. As viewers, we absorb a message: Those who get the best product are the most important. In these ACT-UP materials, we receive a complementary message that African Americans, Latinos, women, and the poor have less intrinsic value, as seen by the quality and quantity of materials and campaigns devoted to their concerns.

In attempting to understand the racial politics of ACT-UP, it is useful to hear the words of one of its strongest supporters, the highly articulate Vito Russo. Speaking in early 1989, his optimism about the ACT-UP strategy for dealing with diversity is evident:

AIDS has touched people of all kinds. And, you know, you might even say that this is an issue which is broader, instead of smaller, than gay rights. Because, first of all it's a huge minority problem which was not recognized until recently. Second of all, when we first instituted ACT-UP it was in response to government inaction, and where we learned most of what we know about government inaction came from the way women have never really been—women's health concerns—have never really been addressed by the medical establishment. How poor people's medical concerns have never been addressed by the medical establishment. And we learned a lot of what we know and what we use in ACT-UP from that.

And so when ACT-UP started, it started as women and men, gay and straight, black and white, in the same room. And there wasn't a necess—I mean it wasn't so much of a necessity for outreach as there was with the gay movement. I mean not that it didn't have to be done, because one of the first things that we did was to form a committee called the Outreach Committee. Because what we wanted to do was, for instance, what we did, and it didn't work so well, unfortunately, was to go into Harlem to black Baptist churches like Abyssinian, to try to talk to ministers about what they were saying to their community. Because we felt that one of the great tragedies of the early years of the epidemic was that the black community did not respond as swiftly and as well as the gay community. The male gay community responded immediately. And that was because there was a tremendous amount of denial in the black community that there was any homosexuality or bisexuality, and a great deal of tension and shame over the issue that if you were saying IV drug users were of the highest risk, why were you also saying that those people were black? Why are they all black? Because there are a lot of white, middle-class people who are IV drug users.

So we had a lot of tension that we, when we went into those churches, we didn't even realize existed, and that was our mistake. Because, first of all, here we were telling these people what to do. And, you know, we learned the lesson that you do not walk into another group's community—especially not into their churches—and try to tell them how to handle a problem. And so it was a huge fiasco, in some ways.

Eventually it worked out, because eventually we worked through channels. I mean Third World members of ACT-UP really preferred to deal with this, number one. It was their community. And number two, we got black politicians, like David Dinkins, who's going to run for mayor in New York this year, and [other] people to be our conduit, so that we could form alliances. And that worked out real well.[40]

Despite his progressive politics, we can see in these comments by Russo a belief that the African American community is less attentive to HIV than is the white gay community. Also in 1989, Russo expressed the correlative belief that if African American community members were really concerned about the politics of HIV care and treatment, they would be at ACT-UP meetings:

I think what you're really talking about is why does not the membership of ACT-UP reflect some of the minority issues that arise from direct membership participation of minorities, etc., etc. And I think that part of the reason for that quite frankly, and I know I can get in a lot of trouble for saying this, is that black people with AIDS and black lesbians and gay men have not done the necessary work in their own community that they need to be doing. And you can't blame everything on racism.

You know, the point is that it's well known that AIDS has not been dealt with extensively in the black community. And part of the reason for that and part of the burden for that and part of the blame for that . . . has to be laid directly on the shoulders of people in the black community who are either gay or have AIDS . . . who have not done the necessary work, and this relates to a traditional problem in minority communities where people are so busy working around issues of racism that they either haven't gotten to issues of homophobia in their own community or are afraid.

See, I think it's a myth. It has yet to be proven to me what is often cited as gospel, which is that machoism and homophobia is much stronger in the black community than it is in other communities. I don't buy it. I think people are just homophobic. I don't think black people are any more homophobic in their community than white people in our community. It's a matter of the degree to which you pursue those issues.

And so when somebody stands up in an ACT-UP meeting and says, "Why don't we have more blacks here?" my response is more often than not, "Yes, racism exists, but that's not the problem here. The problem here is that why aren't these people at this meeting? I can pick up the newspaper and see where 13th Street is and get my fat ass on the subway and come down here. So can you. Why aren't you here?"

And then they'll say, "Well, they're not here because traditionally the gay liberation movement has been a white, middle-class movement, and there's racism and they don't want to be involved with you." And I say, "Well, that's your problem." I mean it's also my problem because I have to fight racism, too. But why aren't hundreds of black people who know that their community is being hit very hard by this disease in that room on Monday nights? They know how to find it. They know when the meetings are. Where are they? And so I'm saying that minority people have to go into their communities and agitate on these issues and they're not. They're just not doing it.

And I don't believe it's because they're afraid that homophobia is much more virulent in their community and like the taboo against homosexuality is allegedly much stronger in the black community. I don't think that's true. I really don't. I think it's just the same as it is everywhere else and they have to learn to fight it. You know? I could be wrong, because they're very church-oriented, and religion plays a big part in that. But they should be agitating in the black churches, in the Baptist churches, they should be getting ministers to speak out on the subject. That's their job, and I don't see it being done.[41]

As these quotations indicate, mobilization of African Americans and other people of color into ACT-UP New York was not successful, though the existing members of the organization did their best to represent the issues of those who were missing.

ACT-UP's issues of identity—as an organization of mostly gay white men who speak concerning issues of gender, race, poverty, and sexuality and advocate for others not extensively represented in their meetings—lead to interesting questions about a movement's organization and mobilization. Clearly the queer culture of ACT-UP is a key to both its appeal to its members and its lack of appeal to others. It is fun to be a part of an organization in which social and cultural transgressions specific to boundaries constructed for your own group are celebrated daily. Thus ACT-UP appealed specifically to gay men and to white gay men at that, because the clothes, the art, the jokes, the language, the political tropes were primarily drawn from New York gay culture. In fact, one might argue that ACT-UP provided an important locus for adult gay socialization and diversification of culture. The organizational focus (stopping the epidemic) is serious and provides legitimation for the entertainment. As Steven Epstein has argued, the culture of gay life has created a kind of ethnic group. With that communal identity and culture one can almost feel in the case of ACT-UP some degree of ethnocentrism that may have blinded members to the different ways that the issues associated with living with AIDS were articulated by others.[42]

Despite its limitations, however, ACT-UP is the most significant direct-action organization to emerge from the epidemic. Its effective incorporation of media, direct action, identity politics, and sophisticated graphics was well suited to its original New York and gay context. It was able to bring in a steady stream of converts to activism, who felt they were actually making a difference in slowing down the epidemic and moving more funds into the search for treatment and cure. In the 1980s New York ACT-UP demonstrated the linkage between cultural forms and organizing strategies by showing just how effective people can be when they work from their strengths. Of course, having access to as much as $600,000 in a good year was a big help, too.

Lessons from the Damned

Contemporary community AIDS organizations face several daunting challenges. One is the difficulty of inter-community and inter-ethnic cooperation. A second issue is staying connected to one's community base, while a third challenge is meeting the consequences of multiple cutbacks in social spending at the same time that the epidemic is spreading. Indeed, a structural perspective concerning disease causation suggests that the direct cause of the AIDS epidemic in the U.S. was economic and social disenfranchisement exacerbated by skewed government spending during the 1980s and 1990s.[1]

Regardless of the emphasis in one's analysis of the broader social institutions, the daily work of preventing HIV transmission and caring for people with AIDS takes place on a local level. Thus an effective response to the epidemic requires both national and local action. As the previous examinations of community-based organizations indicate, race, ethnicity, sexuality, and power—including class-based differences in education, work experience, social contacts, and direct access to money—have an enormous impact on the structure, process, and prioritizing of local AIDS organizing. The results of the distribution of power at the local level can have national repercussions as well, as when the San Francisco AIDS Foundation or New York City ACT-UP influence national policy through the activism of their members or leaders.

Building Community

Just as American society is structured by both overt and unconscious racism, which is enforced and consciously and unconsciously replicated on a large scale, institutional racism also appears in multiple, minute, and obvious ways in grassroots AIDS organizations. We often believe (or hope) that these organizations will be especially sensitive to issues of bias, exclusion, and stereotyping, and in fact their members do seem to be more sensitive than the typical American. If we compare the work of ACT-UP concerning race to that of, say, the American Red Cross, we can appreciate the differences between them.

Given the shared marginalized status of most people with HIV, it makes sense that there would be more sensitivity to oppression, stigma, and stereotyping among those with HIV and those who work in the field. Even if an organizational leader is white and male (and/or straight), he is also associated with a stigmatizing disease. That stigma may have been attached to AIDS and HIV primarily because of the marginalized social status of the majority of people with the disease. But all who are infected are tainted by it; it plays a "master role"—a role that dominates one's perception of others. In the U.S., gender and race also function as master roles, generating distinct behavioral responses in others, regardless of other roles that the individual inhabits, including occupational status.[2] Some authors argue that AIDS will always be stigmatizing, regardless of the identities of the infected, because it is transmitted via sexual activity, and that alone is an important source of stigma.[3]

Despite the values and sensitivities that AIDS awareness generates, survival needs—on both an organizational and a personal level—also drive the members of AIDS organizations. This causes a shortening of focus to the organization's primary activity. The world view of the organization is adopted by the individual employee or member. This socialization to an organizational perspective is necessary if the employee or member of the group is to become a "part" of it. Even if one has different values or opinions than the formal positions of the organization, expression of the "official" point of view is rewarded. As we have seen in all the organizations discussed in this book, the natural tendency of organizations is toward homogeneity, further legitimating the work styles of those already involved.

The ultimate result is that although the agencies, organizations, and groupings can rise to coalition politics in order to affect policy and divide funds, their perspectives are naturally focused on their own needs. Among the organizations that have become large-scale bureaucracies, their internal complexity includes traditional problems of hierarchy, such as organized employee-employer conflict and unionizing, as occurred at the San Francisco AIDS Foundation. Organizations like ACT-UP and the AIDS Foundation, which attempt to become more heterogeneous or to work in heterogeneous coalitions, face the challenge of internal change, especially for the leaders, who have already been rewarded for their "homogeneous" selves.

How are organizations to get past these limitations of culture? Such obvious answers as workshops on diversity seem inadequate because workshops are notorious for being attended by the less powerful in an organization and for creating only superficial change, as happened at the San Francisco AIDS Foundation.

What is needed is more difficult to achieve, but not impossible—the development of interactive communication strategies that reduce intergroup conflict.

This, in turn, relies on understanding the concept of "moral exclusion," which has been defined by the sociologist William B. Gudykunst as occurring "when individuals or groups are perceived as outside the boundary in which moral values, rules, and considerations of fairness apply."[4]

It is common in the U.S. and within the political world of the AIDS movement to emphasize ethnic or racial identity, or class experience, or another specific social category or position as key to cultural identity and difference. Especially with regard to race, our society is organized and divided by these markers, which in turn produce different cultural constructs. Though some groups may retain a sense of being ethnic without having any deep commitment to ethnic social ties and behavior, such purely symbolic ethnicity is a choice only for white ethnics. Non-European Americans do not have such a choice. Other important social identities around which cultures form include gender, disability, age, social class, and sexual orientation. And within the realm of AIDS work a most important social identity is HIV positivity itself. All these social identities are locations or "sites" for the development of cultures and subcultures and, simultaneously, for the development of "intergroup attitudes"—attitudes about people in other groups. Some of the commonly recognized attitudes that hinder communication and reinforce privilege and exploitation are ethnocentrism, prejudice, sexism, and various stereotypes, all of which contribute to the "moral exclusion" of others unlike ourselves.

The concept of moral exclusion is based on the notion of "the stranger" developed by the sociologist Georg Simmel to refer to people who are clearly not members of one's own group. Thus, when the director of the education department at the San Francisco AIDS Foundation argued that lesbians are not at risk of HIV and therefore do not need AIDS education, he was generating a kind of moral exclusion: These women do not need to be "cared for" by an AIDS organization. The comments by Vito Russo concerning the unwillingness of African Americans to come to the Lesbian and Gay Community Center in Chelsea, a gentrified neighborhood in lower Manhattan, and his consequent dismissal of them as "not really interested" in the issues was another form of moral exclusion. Simultaneously, each of the AIDS organizations discussed in this book is constantly fighting against exclusion by the dominant society of those they feel most strongly about: gay people, people of color, drug users, prostitutes, street people. The point here is that moral exclusion can operate on a broad cultural level and also on a small-scale organizational level. In other words, all people with AIDS, may be morally excluded by the dominant society, but also each of the different communities affected by the AIDS epidemic may be itself morally excluded by and morally exclude the others.

Once this phenomenon of moral exclusion is understood, a variety of changes in attitude can occur that facilitate group interaction and communication. Among them are changes in attitude toward other groups, increased complexity of intergroup perceptions, and decategorization; that is, we see people as individuals rather than through stereotyped categories. In many respects, these changes in attitude are reflected in communication skills that can be taught, learned, and cultivated.

There is a useful distinction that can be drawn between "individualist" and "collectivist" cultures, which we can apply to understand the difference between the work atmosphere of the San Francisco AIDS Foundation (and any modern bureaucracy), which assumes an individualist orientation, and that of Cal-PEP, which is more attentive to "family" and a sense of racial community—a collectivist orientation. The members of both organizations live in the same society, but their different locations within that society, primarily due to the salience of race in circumscribing their life choices, create radically different cultural and social experiences for their members, almost as if they lived in different worlds. Although membership in the group "white" is crucial for the majority of players in SFAF (and Prevention Point as well), for whites this identity is unmarked; for this reason, highly differentiated individualism can and does thrive.

It is not easy for individualists and collectivists to understand one another, but this is a skill that can be learned. In a training guide on cross-cultural sensitivity, sociologists Harry Triandis, R. Beislin, and C. H. Hui detail what individualists must understand about collectivists and vice versa. Individualists must:

(a) Recognize that collectivists pay attention to group memberships and use group memberships to predict collectivists' behavior; (b) recognize that when collectivists' group memberships change, their behavior changes; (c) recognize that collectivists are comfortable in vertical, unequal relationships; (d) recognize that collectivists see competition as threatening; (e) recognize that collectivists emphasize harmony and cooperation in the in-group; (f) recognize that collectivists emphasize face (public self-image) and help them preserve their face in interactions; (g) recognize that collectivists do not separate criticism from the person being criticized and avoid confrontation whenever possible; (h) cultivate long-term relationships; (i) be more formal than usual in initial interactions; and (j) follow collectivists' guidance in disclosing personal information.[5]

Their advice for collectivists who wish to interact effectively with individualists (advice an organization like Cal-PEP might follow when dealing with the State of California), is:

(a) Recognize that individualists' behavior cannot be predicted accurately from group memberships; (b) recognize that individualists will be proud of their accomplishments and say negative things about others; (c) recognize that individualists are emotionally detached from their in-groups; (d) recognize that individualists prefer horizontal, equal relationships; (e) recognize that individualists do not see competition as threatening; (f) recognize that individualists are not persuaded by arguments emphasizing harmony and cooperation; (g) recognize that individualists do not form long-term relationships and that initial friendliness does not indicate an intimate relationship; (h) recognize that individualists maintain relationships when they receive more rewards than costs; (i) recognize that individualists do not respect others based on position, age, or sex as much as collectivists; and (j) recognize that the out-groups are not viewed as highly different from the in-group.[6]

It is in the fully aware application of these sorts of learnable skills that we can move beyond our stereotypes, negative expectations of others, and other kinds of rigid thinking that contribute to poor communication across group lines. Elinor Langer, whose work underlies much contemporary training in communication and diversity awareness, calls this "mindfulness."[7] She identifies three characteristics of mindfulness: the creation of new categories, openness to new information, and consciousness of more than one perspective. According to Langer this process does not mean giving up one's ability to judge, but rather being open to a kind of cultural relativism. We must be able to make judgments; but to judge another culture, one must first study it to understand what the actions in it mean.

Cultural relativism—as a way to understand others from different cultural backgrounds—implies an argument for the core values of respect, responsibility, trustworthiness, caring, justice and fairness, and civic virtue and citizenship. These values are grounded in the requirement that we respect others and their ethical views—in other words, moral inclusion.

Moral inclusion as discussed by Gudykunst translates into a set of precepts that can be applied to an organization or a wider collectivity such as a community council:[8]

1. Be committed.
2. Be mindful.
3. Be unconditionally accepting.
4. Be concerned for both ourselves and others.
5. Be understanding.
6. Be ethical.
7. Be peaceful.

Gudykunst argues that community is necessary to make life worth living and to bring peace into the world. This is the individual responsibility of each person, and cultural and ethnic diversity are necessary resources for building community. One person can change a relationship or start the development of a community. Thus, by being open to others, we create new selves for ourselves.

Community cannot exist without conflict. A correlative idea is that if there is to be a community then there must be a way to resolve conflicts. We cannot operate on the reverse notion of resolving all conflicts first before establishing community. Why? Because the community includes the sense of moral inclusion within which conflicts can be resolved. If one insists on moral exclusion it is impossible to resolve conflict.

While these principles may seem idealistic, I believe they offer a vision that can be incorporated by AIDS organizations of all types, regardless of the cultural background, politics, work experience, or goals of the members and leaders. And if precepts such as these are followed, it is possible to create an atmosphere of mutual respect within and among the organizations that will help build a network strong enough to fight both the epidemic and the lack of appropriate services and policies in the broader society.

Even if we solve the problem of sharing power between community groups, and even if each social service or prevention organization is working at its full potential, there will still be a serious problem. Outreach alone cannot prevent AIDS. Local and national policies and cultural practices must also be transformed. Despite fifteen years of education, publicity, and activism, many local governments as well as the federal government still do not view AIDS as a health emergency. Racism, disinterest in the poor, and contempt for gay men have created an atmosphere in which most Americans are willing to passively accept the idea that tens of thousands of people in racially or sexually stigmatized groups will die from a completely preventable disease. The same public evinces little interest in AIDS prevention in these "high-risk" communities unless there is some fear that the epidemic might "spill over"—through blood transfusions, male bisexuality, or female prostitution, for example—into the "wider community," to the "rest of us." One consequence of such attitudes is an emphasis on education and changes in personal behavior for groups at risk without the new social policies that are needed if education is to be effective and if behavioral changes in large segments of the population are to occur.

For example, physicians have been instructed by health departments to advise patients to use condoms,[9] but heterosexual community norms for both men and women are only slightly more supportive of condom use than they were in 1980, and most physicians teach neither technique nor negotiation skills. In American gay communities there has been general acceptance of condom use for anal sex, but there is a growing retreat from using condoms for oral sex. Long-term maintenance of safe sexual practices has proven exceedingly difficult. And young men and women, often only boys and girls, are continually arriving at their first sexual experiences with little sex education, if any, and are unable to avoid HIV exposure. Little permanent change of the sort that can prevent transmission of HIV has occurred in sexual behavior for those who are poor and young. Condoms are expensive, available only in limited locations, and are still being provided to the public without adequate education for safe and effective use. Added to these dangers is the relative powerlessness of women when confronted with male sexual demands.

Effective use of condoms by women and men will require three components: greater availability of free or very low-cost condoms, understandable information on how to use them properly, and the power to use them. All three components require community intervention. In other words, AIDS prevention for those at risk of HIV infection through sexual contact can only be accomplished through basic changes both in community sexual norms and in the economics of preventive health programs.

For those whose risk of AIDS is through dirty needles, only social change will reduce the relative power of the drug economy in American ghettos, barrios, and other poor communities. Such change has been a goal of most poor communities for a number of years, but these neighborhoods, which are highly dependent on government services, have been unable on their own to end the drug trade that weakens them. Their attempts have not been supported by local, state, or federal agencies, and they have not had the power to force that support.

In fact, in some cases government drug policies have run counter to strategies known to help prevent HIV infection. For example, the Reagan and Bush administrations gutted federal support for the already inadequate number of drug rehabilitation programs despite their anti-drug posturing. It took six years after the connection between sharing needles and AIDS transmission became clear for the National Institute on Drug Abuse to consider funding an experimental needle exchange program. This delay did not occur because there was no evidence that such programs can be useful: Evidence to the contrary had already been accumulated in Britain. The United States forbade needle exchange primarily for moral reasons—the same justification that was given to block the provision of condoms in both prisons and high schools, despite their obvious value in these locations. And it was not until 1995 that a federal task force concluded that needle exchange programs could be life-saving, providing an official rationale for government funding for needle exchange. Nevertheless, by 1997, the federal government still had not funded one needle exchange program.

Because of such widespread, federally sanctioned complacency, it seems clear that local community organizing efforts are the most immediate route to saving lives and creating networks of compassion. In preventing AIDS, the second half of the slogan "Think globally, act locally" may well be the most important, as well as the surest route to the global.

The Consequences of Bureaucracy

In order to understand community change and AIDS prevention, it is necessary to have a clear definition of community. A community is a group of people who identify themselves as linked by culture, social organization, language, common experience, or fate. Changing community norms and behavior and gaining access to treatment or education have been the goals of the organizations studied in this book. "Community change" means change within an identified population—encouraging greater willingness to discuss sex and sexuality among Japanese Americans in the San Francisco Bay Area, for instance—as well as change in the relationship between the population and the larger social or political structure in which it exists—such as greater access to treatment for women with HIV.

The degree of control or management of the change process vested in the local community can vary from zero to 100 percent. Hypothetically, at one end of the continuum a community would have no control over the process, and local or national government would attempt to regulate sexuality and drug use rigorously through law and the criminal justice system. State sponsored quarantines of people infected with AIDS represent an extreme form of this approach. At the other extreme, a local community would have a network with economic and political resources and the opportunity and ability to define and pursue health priorities and goals. This latter scenario has been most closely approximated in some gay communities and in scattered ethnic communities. Prevention Point began with complete control over its projects. These community-controlled organizing projects generally survive on donations from within the communities in which they are located, with minor support from foundations or government agencies.

Somewhere in the middle of the empowerment continuum are community-oriented primary health care programs, such as those that work on a block-by-block basis to help neighborhoods define and address health concerns with the support of a medical center or health department.[10] Although this is a promising approach, there are still few AIDS prevention projects of this type.[11]

All of the organizations described in this book began as community-based programs with high levels of local, non-professional, volunteer input. AIDS prevention and service programs of this sort are labor intensive, operate on low budgets, and rely on person-to-person intervention to produce change. Some of these organizations have become professionally based and highly bureaucratic, and all have moved from the most purely community-based model along a continuum toward bureaucratically controlled organizations. Professionally based programs may serve a neighborhood, an ethnic community, or an entire city. They are usually part of an administrative structure that is only indirectly and remotely controlled by the community in which they work. They have less community input in philosophy, daily practice, budgeting, and program planning. They are also often more capital intensive, pay higher salaries, and utilize information transmission (such as media campaigns) or management strategies (such as testing and contact tracing) to bring about behavioral change and social control.

As we have seen in looking at the histories of several AIDS organizations, many programs move from a high level of community involvement to a lower one; few move in the other direction. Figure 7.1 presents an outline of this process. What is the transition that occurs? Where do community-based organizations start and where do they go?

Figure 7.1. Organizational Histories of Community-Based Programs
(Prevention, Education, and Service)

Stage 1: The Grassroots Organization
High community input
Membership organization
Charismatic leadership
Labor-intensive work
Small budgets
Low salaries (if any)
Person-to-person intervention
Extensive use of volunteers
Free services
Group decision-making

Stage 2: Transition to Non-Profit Status
Non-profit incorporation
Board of directors
Reduced community input in policy
Board or staff make all important decisions
More bureaucratic leadership and management
    style
More secondary interventions (media staff do
    more training instead of direct interventions)
    Paid staff grows, directs volunteers

Stage 3: Competition with Established Institutions
(e.g., health departments, public education, Red
    Cross)
Full-scale bureaucracy
Paid staff runs organization
Professional orientation increasingly excludes
    community workers
Reduced use of volunteers or professional
    management of volunteers
Work is capital-intensive
Charges for services
Search for more elite board members who can
    raise greater sums of money

Community-based responses have generally begun in forms that can be characterized as grassroots movements for social change. Whether they are located in a gay community or an African American ghetto or a barrio, whether they emerge from feminist activity or from a meeting of drug rehabilitation providers, grassroots AIDS organizations are usually started by individuals in existing leadership roles within a community, or at least they have a primary connection to the community they are attempting to serve. The grassroots leaders whose stories we have heard in this book are charismatic men and women who have been able to attract and inspire others to join and to volunteer their time and expertise. This is one of the defining characteristics of community-based organizations. For this reason, the organizations usually begin with high community input and group decision-making processes. Most often, they are low-budget organizations, pay small salaries (if any), provide free services, and are extremely labor-intensive.

Typically, these organizations begin on an all-volunteer basis. Gradually they are able to have a small paid staff, but initially the volunteers (or members) outnumber the staff. Partly in response to the opportunity for public and foundation funding, the staff grows and begins to either manage or replace the volunteers. Paid staff becomes increasingly prominent in setting policy and programs and determining the organizational response to external social and political demands as well as internal issues related to the organization's growth and development.

It is at this stage that incorporation as a non-profit usually occurs. The common impetus for this development is the availability of public funding and the demand of funding agencies that fundees have corporate non-profit status. Incorporation requires establishing a board of directors, a new and powerful group to which the staff is officially subordinate. While the organization may have its "stake-holders"—those to whom it feels morally responsible, those who have a "stake" in the organization—the organization's legal boss is its board of directors. Boards of directors can include stake-holders or representatives of the community; nevertheless, this stage of development is usually accompanied by reduced community input into policy and other important decisions of the organization. Board and staff make all the important decisions, and leadership styles grow increasingly bureaucratic and less democratic.

It is not uncommon that when incorporation takes place the paid staff grow in number and become supervisors of the volunteers who were, originally, the heart of the organization. Another common development at this point in growth is that the staff does less direct intervention and more training of others to work in the community. Overall, the immediate effect is that the organization loses its grassroots base and becomes increasingly removed from the community that gave rise to it.

In one form or another, this is the process that all of the organizations described in this book have undergone, though not all to the same degree and not all with the same result. Community investigation or surveillance of an organization can affect the board and the staff composition and policies (as has been the case with both Shanti and SFAF), but essentially the direct power of the community through volunteerism, membership, or participation by self-initiation is lost.

As organizations increase their reliance on public funds, their language and planning process also changes. The fiscal year is increasingly tied to the funding patterns of government agencies and foundations. Organizations begin to use terms like "mission," "goals," and "objectives," with each term having a funding-specific meaning. The mission is supposed to be the organization's vision of its fundamental work. "It should express the heart, not the mind, of the system," as one textbook on organizational development puts it.[12] Goals are the means of achieving the mission. They are measurable, outcome-oriented, relatively short-term products. Objectives are steps by which to achieve the goals. Any grantwriter worth hiring knows that the work of an agency must be translated into goals and objectives. Often the grant application forms have these headings preprinted on them. Some organizations then apply these concepts to their own planning. During the San Francisco AIDS Foundation re-organization process these terms were used over and over again. In addition, they were incorporated into all the planning done by the various departments.

Another concept taken from the for-profit sector and used by both non-profits and funders is the "strategic plan." Strategic plans are future-oriented, have the long-term prosperity of the organization as a goal, utilize extensive organizational resources, and take into account or depend on the external environment in some way.[13]

When the staff of a community-based organization increases in size, the necessity for bureaucratic management grows. Eventually, the organization is run entirely by a paid staff and becomes a full-scale bureaucracy. The professional orientation of the staff increasingly excludes volunteer workers from the community. The work of the organization is no longer labor-intensive; it is capital-intensive and therefore increasingly dependent on funding sources and on charging fees for its services. To ensure the capital it requires to operate, the organization begins to search for elite board members who can aid in raising greater sums of money.

At this point, charismatic leadership becomes less useful and is sometimes harmful to the organization. It is not atypical for community-based organizations that undergo this kind of change to pass through a period of crisis that centers around the need for changes in leadership and leadership style. Among the organizations we have looked at, the struggle that Prevention Point experienced between its volunteers and its new bureaucratic leaders is one example. And though Cal-PEP's original leader remained at the helm, it was only because she accepted the need to disassociate from her "family."

Changes from small- to large-scale and from a volunteer-based to a professionally staffed organization have several correlates in changes in both organizational policy and program. The San Francisco AIDS Foundation's criticism of the ACT-UP demonstration on the Golden Gate Bridge is a classic example.

Although SFAF was founded by community activists, by 1987 its budget was dependent on donations from middle- and upper-class individuals who crossed the bridge on their way to work and thoroughly resented ACT-UP's disturbance of their commute. It was also funded by local government agencies with whom the Foundation required good relations. While staff may have agreed with the concerns of the demonstrators, the organizational commitment to obey the law was paramount.

The movement from charismatically led, community-based organization to professionally led bureaucracy also means that the emphasis on community solidarity and pride that marks the early years of an organization may be replaced by a concern with and striving toward legitimation within a broader, more mainstream value system. Community organizing and self-help models are usually replaced by professional service delivery. This has become a key issue in many AIDS organizations' hiring policies. These staff changes reduce the previously high level of community input. The boards of the AIDS organizations for whom this is true have fewer and fewer members who represent the community and an increasing number of professionals who can assist in fundraising, financial management, legal issues, public relations, and legitimizing the organization in the eyes of mainstream funders and supporters.

What is both ironic and troubling about this process is that even as grassroots AIDS organizations grow and prosper as professionally based service or educational institutions, the original model that they leave behind—community input, organizing, and empowerment—may well be the most promising strategy for AIDS prevention. Most studies of AIDS intervention projects support the theory that community-controlled AIDS prevention works; it is now commonly accepted among public health officials that AIDS-prevention programs should be tailored to the communities in which they are located. This awareness has led to an increased emphasis on materials and events that are culturally appropriate in terms of language, graphics, and content, which are, if possible, disseminated by community members or leaders.

Not even community control can assure that an organization's programs reflect the needs and interests of *all* members of the community it hopes to serve. All too often, as we have seen throughout this book, the needs of women or people of color are left out. Women, for example—and especially women with HIV—are often excluded from planning and managing prevention and service programs. This is partly because women comprise a small proportion of those known to be HIV-infected in the U.S. It can be also attributed to the fact that many HIV-infected women who are active drug users or are seriously ill with AIDS-related infections are incapable of sustaining major involvement in AIDS prevention or care. But the primary reason for women's exclusion is neither lack of numbers, illness, nor apathy: it is the institutionalized sexism and racism that relegate African American women and Latinas to subordinate—and sometimes invisible—positions in organizations ranging from health departments and government administrations to substance abuse programs, AIDS programs, and ethnic advocacy groups. In short, women are still rarely seen or heard.

A consequence of this exclusion is that women's needs take a back seat. Health educators still write brochures asking women to protect their men and their children. Saving their own lives is mentioned last. Further, while men are told to use condoms, women may hear that they should "consider discussing" their use. AIDS residences, food banks, drug programs, and support groups focus on the individual and his or her support network. Provisions to help a mother with her children are often tacked on as delayed afterthoughts.

Communities vary in degree and type of organization, and community organizing must reflect these differences in order to successfully include women. A small migrant labor camp in central Florida may have only rudimentary social institutions, while an East Harlem Puerto Rican neighborhood may be filled with a variety of schools, churches, associations, and familial networks. A neighborhood in San Francisco may have black residents from the American South, Panama, Ethiopia, the Caribbean, as well as third-generation Californians. All three locations—Florida, East Harlem, San Francisco—could have high rates of HIV infection. Community mobilization designed to reach women and to combat the spread of HIV would vary considerably from one location to the other. For example, at the labor camp in Florida, one might work through a health clinic or a prenatal care program, while in San Francisco one might target churches and cultural associations with high rates of participation by women.

Organizing Strategies

Many groups have attempted to change daily life in community settings by organizing the members of the community so that they can have greater control over the basic institutions that determine their lives. The settings for such work range from traditional neighborhood organizing, to labor unions, to movements for ethnic liberation, peace, and women's rights. Some of the best known of the neighborhood organizing work in the United States has been done by Saul Alinsky and others utilizing the techniques he developed.[14] The essence of the Alinsky approach is the identification of community values, traditions, interests, leaders, and factions complemented by organizing people who are spread among the factions but are essentially powerless because they have been divided and unorganized. Alinsky believed that community power was a value in itself. He was less concerned with the specific issues around which the community was organized and more concerned with the development of a powerful organization that could leverage material goals from local or state government. The value of the Alinsky model to those working in AIDS prevention is its flexibility and the wealth of knowledge that has accrued about how to apply it in a variety of situations.

One limitation of the approach is that many local phenomena are controlled by such larger forces as national economic policy and consequent health priorities and funding and are, therefore, not amenable to control by strictly local organizations.[15] Therefore attempts at community organizing in the 1960s and 1970s were built on the techniques of the Alinsky model, but they more often followed a strategy of linkage with similar organizations within a region or, in some cases, nationally. These linking organizations—the Student Nonviolent Coordinating Committee (SNCC), Students for a Democratic Society (SDS), and later, the Association of Community Organizations for Reform Now (ACORN)—combined local community empowerment with national structures. As national organizations, they attempted to develop unified strategies that would produce national social policies in accord with their goals.

There are other models of organizing that also provide lessons for AIDS prevention. Unions, especially within large-scale settings, have achieved important health and safety improvements on the job. And during the 1960s, the National Welfare Rights Organization mobilized thousands of welfare recipients to disrupt welfare offices and insist on increased services.[16] Community-based disease prevention projects, such as the Community Heart Disease Prevention Trials[17] and the National Cancer Institute Community Intervention Trial for Smoking Cessation, changed the habits of thousands.[18] Finally, China, Cuba, and Nicaragua provide models for successful national public health intervention and mobilization. In recent years, a national AIDS prevention program in Uganda has significantly reduced new infections in one of the hardest hit nations in the world.

In the U.S., community organizing is to reach men and women at highest risk for HIV infection and disease, it will need to be located in communities with significant populations of African Americans and Latinos. In 1987, the National AIDS Network surveyed 250 AIDS organizations concerning their participation in AIDS prevention work in minority communities, where the majority of women at risk for HIV infection can be found. Very few organizations served areas with significant minority populations, nor were minorities a significant component of their caseload. This was true for both educational and service organizations.[19] The situation has changed somewhat since the late eighties, but the vast preponderance of resources is still in the hands of organizations controlled by whites.

On the other hand, considerable grassroots community organizing focused on the AIDS epidemic has been done within gay communities. When gay male communities were first denied public resources for AIDS prevention in the early 1980s, they organized themselves to raise private money and to apply political pressure to public agencies. In San Francisco, where the gay community had already established itself economically and politically, this two-pronged approach was effective in reducing viral transmission rates and in providing generally compassionate care.

In 1983, with small grants from the city health department, gay community organizations in San Francisco began major AIDS prevention campaigns. At that time the opinion was publicly expressed around the country—and even within some segments of the gay community—that gay men infected with HIV or at risk of infection were "sex addicts" who had such low self-esteem they believed that they deserved AIDS and were incapable of changing their sexual behavior.[20] However, as a result of community organizing and education, the San Francisco HIV transmission rate associated with gay sexual contact had dropped from 12 percent to two percent by 1985, and the following year it dropped even further. Additionally, the city developed medical and social services that have been cited as national models for both humane and cost-effective care.[21]

A crucial component in the development of the "San Francisco experience," as it has been called, has been the active role of the gay and lesbian community, not only in the provision of services, but also in the exercise of political power. Grassroots organizing of the gay community in the 1970s, especially in the Castro district, resulted in large gay Democratic clubs and the inclusion of both open and closeted gay and lesbian staff throughout the city bureaucracy. When gay community leaders responded to the AIDS epidemic, they utilized the political power of the clubs combined with the community's growing power in the bureaucracy to force the city's health department to respond to the epidemic. When the response was deemed inadequate but no more could be expected at the time, the economic power and the local organizing skills of the gay and lesbian community were turned to the development of community-based alternatives to public services. For example, when the San Francisco Department of Public Health refused to print sexually explicit educational materials, the Harvey Milk Democratic Club and, later, the San Francisco AIDS Foundation printed explicit brochures and posters from their own privately generated funds.

Gay community activists, joined by others concerned about AIDS, raised funds, lobbied, campaigned, and built new organizations. In some cases, they went around the law. Illegal activities included the provision of unapproved medicines, civil disobedience, and individual assistance to those seeking a final escape from pain. These activities were overwhelmingly supported by the gay community in which there was a widespread belief that to survive the epidemic the community must set its own priorities, make its own rules, and generate its own responses.

While the experience of the gay community's AIDS organizing is impressive and in many ways instructive, most ethnic minority communities cannot draw on the financial resources that are available to the predominantly white gay community. Thus far, they have not been able to force state and local governments to respond sufficiently to provide the AIDS prevention, health care, and other services needed in their communities.[22] At the same time, these are communities at risk; they suffer from pervasive poverty, inadequate health services, poor health, a drug epidemic, and a rapidly growing rate of HIV infection and disease.

It is sometimes stated that community organizing to prevent the spread of AIDS in minority communities is unrealistic. Some believe that key elements in the communities at risk are either unable or unwilling to change. Alternatives most commonly suggested are mass media approaches, working with individuals or small groups, or more traditional strategies for social control. The stories of Prevention Point and Cal-PEP indicate that such assumptions can be wrong.

Drug users, a group that comprises a significant proportion of people of color with AIDS, are often described as "unable to change." However, a 1986 New Jersey Health Department study of addicts who were provided with vouchers for treatment indicated that the overwhelming majority of intravenous drug users will seek care and rehabilitation in a therapeutic environment if it is available.[23] In addition, injection drug users in the United States and elsewhere will readily use clean needles if they are available. They will seek out the needles, buy them if they can, and organize their distribution if allowed. For those who wish to avoid HIV by stopping drug use altogether, even in the 1980s President Reagan's AIDS Commission found that the most important obstacle to preventing AIDS among drug users, other than the illegality of holding a clean syringe and other drug paraphernalia, is the lack of adequate treatment programs and lengthy waiting lists for those in existence. Research on women who are drug dependent consistently indicates that a major impediment to their survival and to their ability to change is the lack of woman-appropriate treatment.[24]

Another group that is often scapegoated as unscrupulous HIV infectors of innocent populations are female prostitutes. However, as noted earlier, research conducted by the Centers for Disease Control found no differences in HIV infection rates between prostitutes and other women, despite the fact that prostitutes average many more sexual encounters, including higher rates of intercourse.[25] Those prostitutes who are either infected through sexual contact (sometimes by their steady partners) or through drug use often continue to use condoms with customers. Also, prostitutes on all continents continue to educate themselves about AIDS and develop risk reduction programs that include condom use, drug abuse prevention and safety, education of customers, and legal protection against the scapegoating process. The prostitutes most involved in this work are those who were already organized locally, nationally, and internationally prior to the AIDS epidemic. One consequence of the international nature of the epidemic has been international AIDS meetings and the establishment of communication networks. Prostitutes and prostitute organizers and educators have been welcome at these meetings and have developed new linkages among women in sex work. This has led to the spread of risk-reduction practices among prostitutes globally.

An important contradiction in the attitude of the state toward prostitutes and AIDS is seen in the fact that some prostitute education programs are state funded, as in California and the Netherlands, at the same time that repressive legislation is being passed against prostitutes under the auspices of preventing the spread of the virus. For example, in 1988, the California legislature, by an overwhelming majority, enacted legislation allowing mandatory HIV testing of anyone convicted of prostitution. Previously a misdemeanor, prostitution became a felony if engaged in by an HIV-positive person, regardless of the type of sex act involved. This legislation has had its greatest impact on poor black women, who make up the majority of women infected with HIV and the majority of those arrested for prostitution. They can be forced to undergo non-confidential antibody testing, the results of which will be placed in governmental files. They will also face prison time for the "crime" of having been infected with HIV.

The direct-action model of organizing is another AIDS strategy that has been successful, though it has largely been a gay white effort that has failed to include or adequately represent women or people of color. By 1988, direct-action AIDS-focused organizing projects had spread to more than twenty American cities. The primary focus of ACT-UP continues to be the needs of people who are already infected with HIV, with special emphasis on research and access to new treatments. Matters such as prevention and the development of a political analysis and strategy to combat racism, poverty, or sexism in the provision of services have had a lower priority. Concerns over access to treatment moved many members of ACT-UP to support greater state funding for health care. The most loudly cheered demands at many HIV rallies are those for national health care and better health insurance.

Despite the fact that the AIDS direct-action movement, as epitomized by ACT-UP, has adopted the "correct" rhetoric, it is still not firmly linked to women's issues or to African American, Latino, and other minority communities in its daily practice. Almost all ACT-UP groups are overwhelmingly white. The argument by some white gay men and lesbians that people of color in the U.S. are hard to organize is contradicted by the history of the civil rights movement, the Chicano moratorium, and Wounded Knee, to name only a few civil disobedience and nationalist movements. There have also been many successful union, electoral, economic, and environmental movements by and in communities of color. The AIDS direct-action movement will continue to have only limited value in the struggle against AIDS as long as its base in the African American and Latino communities remains weak.

In addition to the direct-action tradition, political activity focused on AIDS could incorporate more of the lessons learned from the women's health movement of the 1960s and 1970s. The women's "self-help" movement produced some important changes in health care and the analysis of health issues that are relevant to community organizing concerning AIDS. The institutional changes achieved include a dramatic increase in the number of women physicians, a somewhat greater role for women in setting health policy, increased recognition of the right of women to control their own bodies, and the establishment of women's clinics and other women-focused services in both the private and public sectors. Coincident with these changes has been the development of feminist analyses that are based on gender-sensitive socioeconomic models to understand women's health. The self-help movement, epitomized by self-examination and the rise of feminist and collectively run clinics, combined forces with feminist pressure for change in the medical establishment to produce new and reorganized services for women.[26]

In some cities women-focused services provided the base for services and advocacy for women with AIDS. The Women's AIDS Network of the San Francisco Bay Area is an example of a broad-based feminist advocacy network whose members were already involved in direct health services to women prior to the epidemic. The political focus of these and other feminist AIDS organizations throughout the U.S. is on policies that predominantly affect women of color. Still, many of the most active women in the networks are white. The discrepancy is partially due to the tendency of ethnically identified health activists, including women, to work in ethnically identified organizations. Women's AIDS advocacy work through the networks has generally been sensitive to issues of race and class. However, the AIDS epidemic presents feminist health activism with the same challenges of color, class, and world views that must be faced by white gay male activists.

The rise of numerous grassroots organizations in the many communities affected by the epidemic is an extremely important phenomenon that goes beyond the AIDS epidemic. Despite the many racial rifts detailed in this book, AIDS organizations represent a new phase in community organizing. For the first time in a broad-based social movement, difference is being acknowledged and stigmatized identities of many sorts are being given new non-stigmatized value and acceptance. Within the world of AIDS one speaks directly about his gayness, her lesbian identity; his drug use and hers; their time as sex workers; sometimes the details of their sexual experiences and fears. In this movement, the relative newness of the illness, its slow but erratic, fatal and seemingly inevitable course, and the intimate one-on-one circumstances of its transmission combine to reduce the need and value of secrets. The "coming out" model of the gay world and the power that this action lends to the individual is indeed appropriate to AIDS as a social movement (even if it is not "the model" of every gay person's experience).[27] Being "out" or "public" as a representative of a specific group affected by the epidemic is one of the most important sources of a claim to resources by the diverse populations struck by AIDS. Thus, it is precisely those who were most neglected who can now make claims on public resources because of their knowledge of the community that may be carrying a deadly virus. Once the specific stigma of their identity has been confronted, members of these marginalized groups can use the former power of the stigma in a reverse way.

Moreover, within the coalitions and task forces and committees of community oversight, the marginalized meet one another. The divisions of race, class, culture, sexuality, and stigma that both separated them and kept each group to itself are partially overcome through interaction. Common interests, friendships, and understandings not based on ignoring differences but on asserting both difference and common need can emerge and strengthen a movement of those who have been excluded from their share of the country's resources.

By far the overriding lesson to be learned from the organizations that have formed to respond to the threat of AIDS is that community organizing is an essential ingredient in the struggle against the epidemic; and there are still many communities whose members are at high risk that are largely unorganized to protect themselves—African Americans, Latinos, and Native Americans, prison populations and the families of prisoners, teenagers, intravenous drug users, their partners and families, and the sex partners of infected members of a community.

Risk is a relative term: Compared to the residents of Boise, Idaho, San Franciscans are at high risk, while residents of Boise are at higher risk than people in Stanley, Idaho, a much smaller town. But any drug user who has shared unclean needles with strangers in the last ten years is at higher risk than anyone else in the categories just mentioned.

Most people at risk of HIV infection lack the individual economic and social power to effectively protect themselves from the epidemic. Community organizing is a method of mobilizing and involving them in a process of social change that results in heightened ability of the community to control such key aspects of its destiny as providing useful education about HIV transmission and risk. Community organization is not sufficient to prevent AIDS in every individual. But it is a necessary step toward developing the resources, norms, rewards, and sanctions needed within the community to bring about changes in individual behavior. New economic resources, housing, drug treatment centers, battered women's shelters, accessible health services, and child care as well as legal resources will be necessary for communities and individuals to eventually be safe from HIV.

We do not yet know in practice exactly how effective community organizing could be to prevent AIDS. More research is needed in other communities.[28] But we do know that without a diverse approach, which community organizing and community control imply, we are condemning tens of thousands to long, slow deaths from HIV. If we opt for life, let us opt for the conditions that make it possible.

A cautionary note: In the mid-1960s the civil rights movement organized massive numbers of poor African Americans and gained white support for racial change. In response, the federal government launched the "War on Poverty," which was the source of the Model Cities program of the late 1970s and the precursor of various employment programs and the Housing and Urban Development (HUD) block grants of the eighties. These social programs were responses to community pressure and community activism, particularly the civil rights movement. The national responses to HIV, including the community control aspects of such key grants as Ryan White funds, which provide block-grant funding for most AIDS services in the cities most heavily affected, are somewhat analogous to the federal response to the economic and social agenda of the civil rights movement.

What was the result of the War on Poverty and the Model Cities programs? Several studies have demonstrated that these programs led to weakened political mobilization in a variety of ethnic communities, especially among African Americans, while developing a small professional class and an underfunded social service sector. The same phenomena may be recurring as a result of the federal response to the AIDS epidemic. There are numerous parallels in the ways that organizations must compete for funds; the powerful role of universities and their monopolization of research moneys; the initial support and then abandonment of community organizations (often through research projects); the on-going struggle for community control of program content in state-funded projects; and unanswered questions of structural change in the conditions that spread the epidemic.

When communities organize to fight the AIDS epidemic, divisive issues of race, class, and gender must be addressed at the outset if the movement for change is to be successful. Otherwise, organizations will fall apart or will fail to meet their objectives. For instance, greater consumer control of experimental protocols is desirable, but not without guarantees that the consumers include the poor and racial minorities who are the most seriously affected by the disease. Genuine community control will also mitigate against the ever-present possibility that successful organizations will be co-opted, resulting in a greater number of jobs for the few and HIV for the many. Community organizing can also prevent projects being funded because they are the personal pets of particular individuals but do not address the structural conditions that give rise to AIDS in a particular community.

The AIDS epidemic presents a unique organizing opportunity, locally, nationally, and internationally. It is an enormous global health crisis that strikes young adults at the height of their economic potential. It orphans children, affects birth and death rates dramatically, re-organizes hospital utilization, and can wreck economies. Because it is a crisis that crosses divisions of race, gender, class, and sexuality, it can also bring people together across boundaries that usually separate movements for social change. Because the epidemic is international, it has encouraged communication across national and continental borders among many types of activists. Lastly, the epidemic has occurred at a time when major changes are occurring in the international and global economy and in the technology of communication. While some of these changes may have helped spread the epidemic (mass labor migrations and family dislocation, for example), others, such as global computer networking, can help activists communicate directly with their counterparts in other countries in order to develop strategies that respond not only to AIDS but to other social problems that foster its spread.

The International Council of AIDS Service Organizations represents one model of global organizing. The United Nations Global Program on AIDS and the international organizations of women with HIV and people with AIDS who meet at various conference, represent other models. The various AIDS sites on the internet and the World Wide Web provide communication forums, available to those with computer access. But it is unclear how the economics of incorporation of persons from poorer countries and of representation and assuring a voice to the poor themselves will ultimately be solved in this global organizing. The use of scholarships for meeting attendence and transfers of technology are a start, but only a start. Economic globalization is a powerful force in the epidemic that will require a sophisticated response that goes far beyond learning about risk behaviors and personal prevention strategies. Still, the process has begun.

Out of death and difficulty, we can also find the promise of change and the possibility of developing new ways of living together.

Endnotes

Preface
1. A yearly event sponsored by the National Minority AIDS Council, NAPWA, and the AIDS National Interfaith Network and especially attuned to the needs of minority organizations.
2. National Skills Building Conference panel, October 1994.
3. National Skills Building Conference panel, October 1994.
4. National Skills Building Conference panel, October 1994.
5. Randy Shilts, *And the Band Played On* (New York: St. Martin's Press, 1987).

Introduction
1. AIDS Coalition To Unleash Power.
2. California Prevention Education Project.
3. Gay Related Immunodeficiency Disease was a term applied by some physicians and others to describe what was later called Acquired Immune Deficiency Syndrome.
4. Cindy Patton, in *Inventing AIDS*, N.Y.: Routledge, 1990, used the phrase "AIDS service industry" to refer to the professionalized AIDS service organizations which developed in the late eighties.

Chapter 1
1. Ken Plummer, *Telling Sexual Stories: Power, Change, and Social Worlds* (London, New York: Routledge, 1995).
2. Although many other "Women and AIDS" meetings and conferences had been held in the U.S., this was the first with open submissions and review panels on the model of scientific conferences.
3. Recorded talk at HIV Infection in Women Conference, held February 22 through the 24th, 1995 in Washington D.C. WHV95, Tape No. 1, History of the HIV Epidemic in Women, speakers: Patricia Fleming, Maxine Wolfe, Mary Lucey, Katherine Anastos, Rae Lewis-Thornton, Mardge Cohen.
4. For a similar and highly sympathetic view of ACT-UP and its role in the organizing for the 1990 HIV and Women conference, see Gena Corea's *The Invisible Epidemic* (New York: HarperCollins, 1992), in which the story of women and HIV culminates in the activism of the conference.
5. Burkett eventually transformed these and other articles into a book, *The Gravest Show on Earth: America in the Age of AIDS* (Boston: Houghton Mifflin Co., 1995).
6. Tara, talk at AIDS Organizing class, UC Santa Cruz, 2/89.
7. Nancy Stoller Shaw, *California Models for Women's AIDS Education and Services* (San Francisco: San Francisco AIDS Foundation, 1985).
8. Nancy Stoller Shaw, "Preventing AIDS Among Women: The Role of Community Organizing," *Socialist Review,* 100 (Fall 1988): 76-92.

9. Nancy Shaw, "Serving Your Patient with AIDS," *Contemporary OB/GYN*, Vol. 28, No. 4 (October): 141-149.

10. See introduction to Beth E. Schneider and Nancy E. Stoller (eds.), *Women Resisting AIDS: Feminist Strategies of Empowerment* (Philadelphia: Temple University Press, 1995), pp. 1-21.

11. For excellent essays and bibliography on the women's movement since the nineteen sixties, see *Feminist Organizations: Harvest of the New Women's Movement*, ed. by Myra Marx Ferree and Patricia Yancey Martin, (Philadelphia: Temple University Press, 1995).

12. See especially Alice Echols, *Daring to be Bad: Radical Feminism in America, 1967-1975* (Minneapolis: University of Minnesota Press, 1989), for an analysis of the radical side of 1970s feminism.

13. This approach, which obscures the activity of those who do not command major amounts of resources and media, is repeated in the histories of many movements, where the roles of the poor, the oppressed, and the companions of the powerful are repeatedly denigrated or made invisible because they have produced fewer material records of their role (fewer books, films, newspapers, paintings) which are easily accessible to historians and journalists of dominant classes and races. They are then proclaimed non-existent as activists and creators.

14. See Barbara Epstein, "Lesbians Lead the Movement," *Out/Look* (Summer 1988): 27-32.

15. It is interesting that when straight, white men write the history of the seventies, again and again they record the death of "the movement." What movement do they mean? Perhaps it is "their" movement (the anti-war movement built on the civil rights movement) which was moribund. Of the active movements of the seventies, which they did not lead, they seem to see little, perhaps because they were not in their center. Feminism, gay rights, movements in Latino and Native American communities, the rise of mass-based anti-nuclear activism, and environmentalism are sometimes labeled "identity politics" and defused into cultural politics. Defining these movements as being primarily about identity gives the incorrect impression that they are simply about the assertion of community and not about structural issues.

16. John D'Emilio, "The Gay Community After Stonewall," in John D'Emilio (ed.), *Making Trouble: Essays on Gay History, Politics and the University* (New York: Routledge, 1992); Estelle Freedman and John D'Emilio, *Intimate Matters: A History of Sexuality in America* (New York: Harper and Row, 1988).

17. Sarah Hoaglund, *Lesbian Ethics* (Palo Alto: Institute of Lesbian Studies, 1988).

18. It has been argued by recent theorists that female development moves in the direction of a relational orientation in contrast to male developmental emphasis on individuation and separation. Carol Gilligan, for example, argued that within Western culture, male moral development has emphasized an ethic of justice, while that of women has greater emphasis on caring (*In a Different Voice: Psychological Theory and Women's Development* [Cambridge, MA: Harvard University Press, 1982]).

19. See Beverly Burch, "Psychological Merger in Lesbian Couples: A Joint Ego Psychological and Systems Approach," *Family Therapy*, 9(3) (1982): 201-277; Jo Ann Krestan and Claudia Bepko, "The Problem of Fusion in the Lesbian Relationship," *Family Process*, 19(3) (1980) 277-289; and Sondra Smalley, "Dependency Issues in Lesbian Relationships," *Journal of Homosexuality*, 14(1/2) (1987): 125-136.

20. Cf. Melissa A. McNeill, *Who Are "We"? Exploring Lesbian Involvement in AIDS Work* (Smith College School of Social Work, Master's Thesis, 1991).

21. The alert reader will note the parallelism between my typology and recurrent value constructs concerning appropriate women's roles: traditionalism, liberal feminism, socialist feminism (coalition building), and radical/separatist/lesbian feminism. Such constructs are widespread and associated with a variety of (sub)cultures, social systems and activist organizations.

22. By this term I mean people who received their primary income from AIDS activities and who meet the sociological definition of a professional, someone whose primary value is in his or her education and receives honorific payment.

23. McNeill, *Who Are "We"?*, p. 50.

24. Interestingly, in 1992, the notion that lesbians have little risk from AIDS and are suffering from "virus envy" resurfaced in England, where it was evident in posters from the Terrence Higgins Trust which proclaimed that "Oral sex is very low risk, so throw away those dental dams." Lesbian inventors of the posters claimed that safe sex emphasis for lesbians was the result of a negative attitude toward sex combined with a desire for more recognition.

25. McNeill, *Who Are "We"?*

26. Katy Taylor of the New York Human Rights Commission (1989 interview).

27. "About 142,000 American women develop [breast cancer] each year and 43,000 die of it. Only lung cancer causes more cancer deaths among American women." "Childhood X-Rays Linked to Breast Cancer Risk," *New York Times,* Nov. 9, 1989: B22, referring to an article in the New England Journal of Medicine for 11/9/89. (Reference cited by separatists in 1989 and 1990.)

28. Jackie Winnow, "Lesbians Working on AIDS: Assessing the Impact on Health Care for Women," *Out/Look,* 5 (1989): 10-18.

29. McNeill, *Who Are "We"?*, p. 55.

30. Harm reduction theory is the analytic approach adopted by advocates of needle exchange to provide a theoretical basis for their work. The starting point of this approach is to "reduce harm" by whatever means possible, without engaging in a moral discourse concerning the potentially dangerous action.

Chapter 2

1. A group of gay men in San Francisco who dress as nuns in a camp style with equally camp names.

2. Cleve Jones, National Skills Building Conference, 1985.

3. *Alice Reports,* Alice B. Toklas Democratic Club, May 1985, p. 1.

4. See Charles Perrow and Mauro F. Guillen, *The AIDS Disaster: The Failure of Organizations in New York and the Nation* (New Haven: Yale University Press, 1990).

5. Executive directors of the SFAF have included Rick Crane (7/82-2/84), Ed Power (Acting, 2/84-5/84), Jim Ferels (5/84-4/85), Mitch Bart (Acting, 4/85-9/85), Tim Wolfred (9/85-89), and Pat Christen (89-).

6. Bob Bolan, M.D., *San Francisco AIDS Foundation Annual Report,* 1985, p. 1.

7. SFAF *Annual Report,* 1985.

8. "Staff comments on diagnosis," mimeo, n.d.

9. At the same time, in NYC this issue had also come to the fore in the Gay Men's Health Crisis (GMHC), where a minority caucus had been formed and was complaining of

a lack of sensitivity throughout their organization. At the time of the GMHC complaints, the AIDS caseload for NYC was 53 percent black and Hispanic, yet there were no people of color in the GMHC administration and program planning for women ignored drug abuse, the number one cause of female infections in the city (Colin Robinson, "53% is no Minority," *The Volunteer,* #3:7, n.d., p. 1).

10. The Sherover-Marcuse model incorporates an argument that diverse groups share the common experience of oppression as children; that we are taught systems of oppression in daily life; that we can be privileged in one dyadic system (e.g., racism) and targeted in another (e.g., sexism). An "unlearning racism" workshop attempts to teach the model and give skills for "unlearning" the learned behaviors which maintain the system.

11. Decision-making solution team, "Milestones," mimeo, n.d. (est. date, 9/86).

12. SFAF *Annual Report,* 1992, p. 1.

13. In February, 1985, almost one-third of calls were from women (male-993; female-325). SFAF Hotline monthly statistics, 2/85.

14. Nancy Stoller Shaw, field notes, 3/14/85.

15. There were six groups specifically for women and specifically about AIDS: the eight-week Support Group for Women at Risk at the AIDS Health Project; a Women Concerned about AIDS group for those "working in the field, women at risk, and with friends or family with AIDS" at the Pacific Center in Berkeley (an agency which primarily served the lesbian and gay community at the time); the Informal Network of women exposed to AIDS and the Women's Program for resources, referrals, information, research updates at the Foundation; a Drop-in Support Group for women whose sexual partner has been diagnosed with AIDS at Shanti; and the Women's AIDS Network, which was primarily for providers and advocates. "Current Support Groups . . . ," SFAF, April, 1985.

16. The HIV anti-body test was still being developed. "Risk" language still used the term "AIDS."

17. "Rehabilitation Resources for Women with I.V. Drug Dependencies," SFAF, 2/1/85 (xerox).

18. Shaw to Starkweather, 8/20/85.

19. Anne Semans, "People with AIDS Living in Streets, Commission Told," *Bay Area Reporter,* 2/13/86: 4.

20. Schietinger to Soler, 3/20/86; Shaw to Soler, 4/29/86.

21. Lawrence Wallack, Lori Dorfman, David Jernigan, and Makani Themba, *Media Advocacy and Public Health* (Newbury Park: Sage, 1993).

22. Future ethnic community research within the city was handled primarily by Polaris Research, a black-owned firm, and by other ethnic-identified agencies.

23. Jackson Peyton to Sam Puckett, "Re: Het Brochure," 10/24/86 (xerox).

24. The famous *Cosmopolitan* magazine scandal was about this exactly, when a psychiatrist wrote an article suggesting that heterosexual HIV transmission was a myth and that such transmission occurred in Africa because the men had sex "like rape" there, unlike sex in the U.S. Demonstrations against *Cosmo* and the psychiatrist's comments were documented in the video *Doctors, Liars and Women* by Jean Carlomusto and others (1989).

25. Theodore W. Allen, *The Invention of the White Race* (London/New York: Verso, 1994).

26. Phillip Brian Harper, "Eloquence and Epitaph: Black Nationalism and the

Homophobic Impulse in Responses to the Death of Max Robinson," *Social Text*, 28, 9.3 (1991) pp. 68-86.

27. This aspect of gay sexuality is explored in the work of Richard Fung, Kobena Mercer, Lee Edelman, and others. See Fung's "Looking For My Penis," in *Bad Object Choices* (ed.), *How Do I Look?* (Seattle: Bay Press, 1993), pp. 145-169. See also Mercer's "Looking for Trouble," in Henry Abelove, Michele Aina Barale, and David M. Halperin (eds.), *The Lesbian and Gay Studies Reader* (New York: Routledge, 1993), pp. 350-359. And see Edelman's "The Part for the (W)hole: Baldwin, Homophobia, and the Fantasmatics of 'Race,'" in Lee Edelman (ed.), *Homographesis* (New York: Routledge, 1994), pp. 42-75.

28. Toni Morrison, *Playing in the Dark* (Cambridge, MA: Harvard University Press, 1992), pp. 9-10.

29. See further, Ruth Frankenberg's *White Women, Race Matters: The Social Construction of Whiteness* (Minneapolis: University of Minnesota Press, 1993), as well as essays in Steven Gregory and Roger Sanjek (eds.), *Race* (New Brunswick: Rutgers University Press, 1994), esp. those by Sacks, Rodriguez, and Trouillot.

30. An exceptionally clear presentation of the naturalization of race is found in Howard Winant's *Racial Conditions: Politics, Theory, Comparisons* (Minneapolis: University of Minnesota Press, 1994). For an interesting historical look at the construction of racism, examining its social, economic, political, and regulatory reproductive components, (see Allen, 1994), in which the author compares the racialization of Irish-British relations with the development of the American black race.

31. This issue of the regime of the normal, a Foucaultian concept, is at the center of the debates concerning a gay and lesbian scholarship and identity, as opposed to a "queer" perspective, in which the argument is presented that "queer" is, by definition, anti-normal and, for some, perhaps better than normal. See Michael Warner's "Introduction" to his *Fear of a Queer Planet: Queer Politics and Social History* (Minneapolis: University of Minnesota Press, 1993), p. xxvi; also the articles by Donna Penn ("Queer: Theorizing Politics and History") and Henry Abelove ("The Queering of Lesbian/Gay History") in *Radical History Review: Queer*, Vol. 62 (Spring 1995): 22-44 and 44-58.

32. Norm Nickens, "AIDS and Ethnic Minorities," *Alice Reports*, San Francisco, Alice B. Toklas Lesbian/Gay Democratic Club-Club Edition. May 1985, p.1.

33. Nancy Shaw, "Monthly Report," Education Department, SFAF, June 1985.

34. Shaw to Stroud, 5/15/85.

35. Stroud to Shaw, 6/5/85.

36. Donald O. Lyman, cover letter to "Request for Proposals for the Acquired Immunity Deficiency Syndrome (AIDS) Pilot Projects for Treatment and Counseling Services for Underserved Minority Populations (October 1986)," 11/5/86 (xerox).

Chapter 3

1. Field work for this chapter was conducted by Christine Wong in 1993. Interviewees included Bart Aoki, Rene Astudillo, Kevin Fong, Ginny Bourassa, David Cho, Vi Huynh, James Naritomi, Ippei Yasuda, Fatima Angeles, Vincent Sales, Robert Bernardo, Kyle Monroe-Spencer, and Steve Lew. All interviews were conducted by Christine Wong.

2. J. Naritomi, Interview (Japanese Community Youth Council, May 7, 1993).

2a. Steve Lew, Interview (Gay Asian Pacific Alliance Community HIV Project, 5/28/93).
3. Sales, Interview (Asian AIDS Projects, May 10, 1993).
4. Lew, 1993.
5. Sales, 1993.
6. D. A. Lee and K. Fong, "HIV/AIDS and the Asian and Pacific Islander Community," Unpublished SIECUS Report (February/March 1990).
7. Vi Huynh, Interview (Chinatown Youth Center, 5/3/93).
8. Lee and Fong, 1990.
9. Interview, 2/93.
10. B. Aoki, Interview (Asian American Recovery Services, 4/19/93).
11. Asian/Pacific AIDS Coalition (A/PAC), 1993.
12. Lee and Fong, 1990.
13. B. Aoki, C. P. N. Ngin, B. Mo, and D. Y. Ja, "AIDS Prevention Models in the Asian American Communities," in V. M. Mays, G. W. Albee, and S. F. Schneider (eds.), *Primary Prevention of AIDS: Psychological Approaches* (Newbury Park, CA: Sage, 1989), pp. 290-308.
14. Lee and Fong, 1990.
15. As early as 1991, the rapid spread of HIV in southeast Asia was predicted by Jonathan Mann (former director of the United Nations' AIDS program) in the *International Journal of Health Services*. ("Global AIDS: Critical Issues for Prevention in the 1990s,") Vol. 21:3, 553-559.
16. *Mid City Numbers: A Monthly Bulletin of AIDS-Related Statistics,* Vol. 8, No. 1 (April 1995).
17. San Francisco Department of Public Health, "AIDS Monthly Surveillance Report" (3/31/93).
18. San Francisco Department of Public Health, 1993.
18a. Raw numbers and per capita rates can tell very different stories. For example, in 1997 the San Francisco Department of Public Health estimated that 8.3% of Native Americans in the city were HIV-positive. This was the highest rate per capita for any ethnic group, including whites, who had the next highest rate (5.4%). However, because Native Americans consituted less than 1% of the city's population, the total number of cases among them would have been low.
19. A/PAC, 1993.
20. Sales, 1993.
21. *Ibid.*
22. *Ibid.*
23. Sales, 1993.
24. Lydia Gomez, Maria Rosario G. Araneta, and J. Geaga, *AIDS Knowledge, Attitudes, Beliefs, and Behaviors in a Household Survey of Filipinos in San Francisco.* Volume 1: "Findings, Summary, and Conclusions" (A Joint Project of the San Francisco Department of Public Health AIDS Surveillance Office, The Asian American Health Forum, and the Filipino Task Force on AIDS-Northern California, 1990).
25. Aoki, 1993.
26. Davis Ja, Kerrily Kitano, and Aaron Ebata, *AIDS Knowledge, Attitudes, Beliefs, and Behaviors in a Household Survey of Chinese in San Francisco* (San Francisco Department of Public Health, 1990).
27. Huynh, 1993.

28. Davis Ja, Kerrily Kitano, and Aaron Ebata, *AIDS Knowledge, Attitudes, Beliefs, and Behaviors Study of the Japanese Community* (San Francisco Department of Public Health, 1990).
29. I. Yasuda, Interview (Japanese Community Youth Council, 5/7/93).
30. Keriji Murase, Susan Sung, and Vu Duc Duong, *AIDS Knowledge, Attitudes, Beliefs, and Behaviors Study of San Francisco Southeast Asian Communities* (San Francisco Department of Public Health, 1990).
31. Monroe-Spencer, 1993.
32. Yasuda, 1993.
33. Yasuda, 1993.
34. Yasuda, 1993.
35. Lew, 1993.
36. Lew, 1993.
37. Angeles, Interview, (Filipino AIDS Education Project, 2/19/93).
38. San Francisco *Sunday Examiner and Chronicle*, 1993.
39. Huynh, 1993.
40. Lew, 1993.
41. Asian/Pacific AIDS Coalition, 1993.
42. Yasuda, 1993.
43. *Bay Area Reporter*, 1993.
44. *Bay Area Reporter*, 1993.
45. K. McLaughlin, "Low AIDS Rates Gave Asians False Confidence," *San Jose Mercury News*, August 31, 1992; J. Mann, D. Tarantola, and T. Netter, *AIDS in the World* (Cambridge: Harvard University Press, 1992).

Chapter 4
1. Thanks to Wendy Chapkis, who co-wrote an earlier version of this chapter. For further exploration of her ideas, see her book, *Live Sex Acts: Women Performing Erotic Labor* (New York: Routledge, 1997).
2. Pricilla Alexander, "Sex Workers Fight Against AIDS: An International Perspective," in Schneider and Stoller, 1995.
3. See further John D. McCarthy and Mayer N. Zald, *The Trend of Social Movements in America: Professionalization and Resource Mobilization* (Morristown, NJ: General Learning Press, 1973).
4. My own field data have been supplemented by interviews conducted by Wendy Chapkis and are further informed by analyses which have emerged from work on feminist debates on pornography and prostitution.
5. Gloria Lockett Interview, 1996.
6. Lockett, 1996.
7. "Postmodernists claim the construction and choice of one story over others is not governed by a relation to truth, but by less innocent factors. These ultimately include a will to power partially constituted by and expressing a desire *not* to hear certain other voices or stories." (Jane Flax, *Thinking Fragments* [Berkeley: University of California Press, 1990], p. 195).
8. Sarah Wynter of WHISPER, for instance, defines prostitution as "enforced sexual abuse under a system of male supremacy" in Frédérique Delacoste and Priscilla Alexander, *Sex Work: Writings by Women in the Sex Industry* (San Francisco: Cleis

Press, 1987), p. 268
9. Sydney Biddle Barrows, *Mayflower Madam: The Secret Life of Sydney Biddle Barrows* (New York: Arbor Press, 1986).
10. Interview with Santa Cruz, CA Sheriff Al Noren, 2/25/88.
11. "Reformed Prostitutes Take to the Streets to Help Their Sisters." *San Francisco Chronicle.*
12. Priscilla Alexander, a co-founder of Cal-PEP, notes in "Prostitutes Prevent AIDS, a Handbook for Health Educators," that the very ability of prostitutes' organizations to raise funds for their outreach work might be compromised by the necessary political lobbying that they feel compelled to do. Hence Alexander suggests: "goals related to police practices involve lobbying, in some cases, and might best be carried out by other organizations" to protect the non-profit status as well as the legitimacy established by adopting the identity of health outreach workers not political activists.
13. "Pros: the Newsletter of the [Australian] Prostitutes' Rights Organization," June 1989.
14. Alexander, xerox, 1996.
15. Valerie Jenness, *Making It Work: The Prostitute's Rights Movement in Perspective* (New York: Aldine de Gruyter, 1993).
16. *San Francisco Chronicle,* August 17 and 19, 1993.
17. Field notes, 8/31/93. As these notes indicate, I was sometimes an active participant in the processes I was studying.
18. Lockett, 2/14/93.

Chapter 5
1. Daniel Goleman, "Researcher Kills Myth of Shared Syringes," *New York Times,* 9/20/95.
2. *Ibid.*
3. Don C. Des Jarlais, Samuel R. Friedman, and William Hopkins, "Risk reduction for the Acquired Immunodeficiency Syndrome among intravenous drug users," *Annals of Internal Medicine,* Vol. 103 (1985): 755-759.
4. Samuel Friedman, Don C. Des Jarlais, J. L. Sotheran, Jonathan Garber, Henry Cohen, and Donald Smith, "AIDS and self-organization among intravenous drug users," *The International Journal of the Addictions,* 22(3) (1987): 201-219.
5. In my own work, looking across communities, cultures, classes, and racial categorizations at the responses of different groups to the epidemic, I have found Friedman's work especially inspiring, because it starts with all groups on an equal par, rejecting stereotypes and stigmatization. My writing on Prevention Point and my general attempts to apply a model which asks about social context, including legality, access to resources, gender, and racial/cultural background and experience to explain organizing strategies, have been strongly influenced by Friedland's own resistance to the psychological, medical and biological determinism so rampant in the "scientific" literature about HIV.
6. Early studies of the British exchanges were reported by Russell Newcombe in "The Liverpool Syringe Exchange Scheme for Drug Injectors: Initial Evidence of Effectiveness in HIV Prevention" (summary paper), First International Conference on the Global Impact of AIDS, March 1988; Gerry Stimson, "Injecting Equipment Exchange Schemes in England and Scotland," in R. J. Battjes and R. W. Pickens (eds.), *Needle Sharing Among Intravenous Drug Abusers: National and International Perspectives,* NIDA Research Monograph 80, 1988, pp. 89-99; and Geoff Rayner and

Karen Gowler, "The Lessons of AIDS," *New Society,* April 8, 1988: 10-12.

7. Luis Kemnitzer, interview, 8/95.

8. Moher Downing, George Clark, Marcie Rein, and Delia Garcia, "Establishing a Street-Based Needle Exchange: Prevention Point's Experience," Prevention Point Research Group, 1991.

9. See Brooke Grundfest Schoepf's chapter on action research in Zaire in Schneider and Stoller, for a general discussion of the interactive nature of this sort of research where ethnographers or other social scientists work with local residents to design interventions or social change strategies.

10. Moher Downing, et al., p. 9.

11. Peter Lurie and Arthur Reingold, *The Public Health Impact of Needle Exchange Programs in the United States and Abroad,* Vol. 2, Centers for Disease Control and Prevention, Oct. 1993, pp. 101-115.

12. From Kemnitzer files.

13. Lori Olszewski, "S.F. Volunteers Giving Addicts Clean Needles," *San Francisco Chronicle,* 3/13/89: A1.

14. "Needle Swap Urged," *San Francisco Chronicle,* 3/22/89: A1.

15. Anonymous, "A Clash Over Needles," *San Francisco Chronicle,* 3/23/89: A4.

16. Naomi Gray, "Needle Exchange: An Opposing View," mimeo, nd. (submitted to the Health Department, summer, 1989).

17. Heidi Evans and Mike Santangelo, "O'C Blasts Addict Plan," *Daily News,* 2/1/88.

18. See Cherni L. Gillman, "Genesis of New York City's Experimental Needle Exchange Program: A Denigrated Group Makes it to the Government Agenda," Narcotic and Drug Research, Inc., 1989 (xerox) for a thorough account of the beginnings of needle exchange programs in New York City in 1988.

19. Lurie and Reingold, pp. 13-28.

20. Sheigla Murphy, Lynn Wenger, and Margaret Kelley, "Community Health Works: An Ethnographic Evaluation of San Francisco's Needle Exchange: Final Report to NIDA" (San Francisco: Institute for Scientific Analysis, 1996).

21. *Ibid,* p. 44.

22. Prevention Point Retreat minutes, 5/19/90.

23. Interview, Alex Kral (AK), 11/95.

24. AK interview, 11/95.

25. Kral's phrasing. Interview, 11/95.

26. AK interview. 11/95

27. AK interview, 11/95.

28. AK interview, 11/95.

Chapter 6

1. See Frances Fox Piven and Richard A. Cloward's approach to the cycling of movements in *Poor People's Movements: Why They Succeed, How They Fail* (New York: Pantheon Books, 1977).

1a. Steven Epstein's *Impure Science: AIDS Activism, and The Politics of Knowledge,* (Berkeley: University of California, 1996), provides the best account to date of ACT-UP's role in changing biomedical research practice.

2. For introductions to Foucault's thinking and its relevance to queer theory and gay organizing, see Michel Foucault, *The History of Sexuality: An Introduction, Vol. 1,* trans. by Robert Hurley (New York: Vintage, 1990); Hubert L. Dreyfus and Paul

Rabinow, *Michel Foucault: Beyond Structuralism and Hermeneutics*, 2nd Edition, (Chicago: University of Chicago Press, 1982); and especially David Halperin, *Saint Foucault: Towards a Gay Hagiography* (New York: Oxford University Press, 1995). Halperin emphasizes Foucault's own political engagement, which included participation in street battles with French police, and elaborates on concepts in Foucault's work that are especially relevent to AIDS activism, such as the notion of the body as a site of political struggle, the use of sexuality as a form of disciplinary regulation by the state, the notions of freedom and resistance as internal to power, and the role of discourse in the maintenance of power relations. If the established rules of discourse maintain power relations, disruption of those rules can also disrupt power relations.

2a. See Josh Gamson's analysis in "Silence, death, and the invisible enemy: AIDS activism and social movement 'newness,'" in *Social Problems*, Vol. 36, #4 (Oct. 1989), pp. 35–368.

3. "In this year [1982], Gay Men's Health Crisis was officially founded by Nathan Fain, Dr. Lawrence Mass, Paul Popham, Paul Rapoport, Edmund White, and me. In a retrospect that, sadly, only Larry, Edmund, and I are still alive to share, this year of 1982 and, for me, the year or so following, was an inspirational time." (Larry Kramer, *Reports from the Holocaust: The Making of an AIDS Activist* [New York: St. Martin's Press, 1989], p. 22). See also Philip M. Kayal, *Bearing Witness: Gay Men's Health Crisis and the Politics of AIDS* (Boulder, CO: Westview Press, 1993).

4. Kramer, *Reports*, p. 32.

5. Indicating that GMHC and Kramer were already knowledgeable about the inside workings of the government.

5a. Kayal's book supports this point.

6. "An Open Letter to Richard Dunne and Gay Men's Health Crisis," New York Native, #197 (1/26/87) (pp. 100-115 in *Reports from the Holocaust*).

7. Vito Russo Interview 10/2/89.

8. *Ibid.*

9. *Ibid.*

10. Terence Kissack, "Freaking Fag Revolutionaries: New York's Gay Liberation Front, 1969-1971," *Radical History Review: The Queer Issue*, #62 (Spring 1995): 104-134.

11. Kramer, pp. 37-8.

12. Russo, Class Talk, University of California, Santa Cruz, 2/89.

13. Douglas Crimp and Adam Rolston, *AIDS Demographics* (Seattle: Bay Press, 1990), p. 28.

14. Kramer, 1989.

15. Russo, Class Talk, 2/89.

16. *Ibid.*

16a. See Epstein's account, 1996.

17. Statistics cited by Abigail L. Halcli in "AIDS, Anger, and Activism: A Conceptual Analysis of ACT-UP as a Mixed Mode Social Movement Organization," presented at the annual meetings of the American Sociological Association, 1992; source identified as New York City and San Francisco chapters of ACT-UP.

18. Thanks to Jason Welle for his excellent research on the chronology of ACT-UP demonstrations.

19. Douglas Crimp, with Adam Rolston, *AIDS Demographics* (Seattle: Bay Press, 1990), p. 33. The authors were both members of ACT-UP at the time the book was prepared.

20. *Ibid*, p. 34.

21. *Ibid*, p. 35
22. *Ibid*, p. 44
23. New member packet, 10/16/89 meeting.
24. Crimp and Rolston, p. 10.
25. *Ibid*, p. 72.
26. *Ibid*, p. 39.
27. *Ibid*, p. 42.
28. *Ibid*, p. 46.
29. *Ibid*, p. 16.
30. *Ibid*, pp. 48, 49.
31. *Ibid*, p. 54.
32. *Ibid*, p. 55.
33. *Ibid*, pp. 66-69.
34. Richard Meyer, "This Is To Enrage You: Gran Fury and the Graphics of AIDS Activism," in Nina Felshin (ed.), *But Is It Art?* (Seattle: Bay Press, 1995), p. 62.
35. Meyer, pp. 64-65.
36. An art auction on Dec. 3 1989 raised $314,000 (*New York Native*, 12/18/89). The auction was organized by ACT-UP member Peter Staley, born to wealth in a Philadelphia Main Line family.
37. Interview, 10/2/89.
38. Crimp and Rolston, p. 30.
39. The ACT-UP/New York Women and AIDS Book Group (Boston: South End Press, 1990).
40. Russo, Class Talk, winter, 1989, p. 7.
41. Russo Interview, 10/2/89.
42. Steven Epstein, "Gay Politics, Ethnic Identity: The Limits of Social Constructionism," *Socialist Review*, Vol. 17, No. 3 & 4 (May-Aug., 1987): 9-54.

Chapter 7

1. Structural analysis of disease causation has been argued by Sylvia Noble Tesh, *Hidden Arguments: Political Ideology and Disease Prevention Policy* (New Brunswick, NJ: Rutgers, 1988).
2. A role which dominates the perceptions of others. In the U.S. gender and race also function as master roles, generating distinct behavioral responses in others, regardless of other roles which the individual inhabits, e.g. an occupational role.
3. This argument is developed in Allan Brandt's *No Magic Bullet: A Social History of Venereal Disease in the United States Since 1880* (New York: Oxford University Press, 1985).
4. S. Optow, "Moral Exclusion and Injustice: An Introduction," *Journal of Social Issues*, 46(1): 1-20. I will be drawing heavily on the work of William B. Gudykunst, who in turn owes much of his perspective to the work of Elinor Langer.
5. Advice for individualists: from Harry Triandis, R. Brislin, and C. H. Hui, "Cross-cultural Training Across the Individualism-Collectivism Divide," *International Journal of Intercultural Relations*, 12(1988): 269-289.
6. Triandis, Brislin, and Hui.
7. Elinor Langer, *Mindfulness* (Reading, MA: Addison-Wesley, 1989).
8. William B. Gudykunst, *Bridging Differences: Effective Intergroup Communication*, 2nd ed. (Thousand Oaks, CA: Sage, 1994), pp. 226-228.

9. C. Horsburgh, et al., "Preventive Strategies for Sexually Transmitted Diseases for the Primary Care Physician," *JAMA*, Vol. 258, No. 6 (August 14, 1987): 815-821.

10. See the following for some examples of this type of community-oriented primary health care: D. Werner and B. Bower, *Helping Health Workers Learn* (Palo Alto, CA: Hesperian Foundation, 1982); and Richard Couto, *Streams of Idealism and Health Care Innovation* (New York: Teachers College Press, 1982).

11. National AIDS Network, "AIDS Education and Support Services to Minorities: A Survey of Community-Based AIDS Service Providers" (Washington, D.C., 1987).

12. Rodney W. Napier and Matti K. Gershenfeld, *Groups: Theory and Experience* (Boston: Houghton Mifflin, 1993), p. 204.

13. Napier and Gershenfeld, p. 205.

14. S. Alinsky, *Reveille for Radicals* (New York: Vintage, 1969).

15. See Robert Fisher and Joseph M. Kling's "Leading the People," *Radical America*, Vol. 21, No. 1 (February 1988), for a comparison of Alinsky's strategy with that of the American Communist Party, which emphasized overt ideological leadership in local activism.

16. Frances Fox Piven and Richard A. Cloward, *Poor People's Movements* (New York: Vintage, 1979).

17. J. Farquhar, et al., "The Stanford Five-City Project: An Overview," in Joseph D. Matarazzo (ed.), *Behavioral Health: A Handbook of Health Enhancement and Disease Prevention* (New York: J. Wiley & Sons, 1984) and J. Farquhar, et al. "Community Education for Cardiovascular Health," *Lancet*, No. 1 (1977): 1192-1195.

18. A. McAlister, "Community Studies of Smoking Cessation and Preventions," in *Health Consequences of Smoking for Chronic Obstructive Lung Disease: A Report of the Surgeon General* (Washington, D.C.: Public Health Service, 1984).

19. National AIDS Network, "AIDS Education and Support Services to Minorities."

20. See P. Harder, et al., *Evaluation of California's AIDS Community Education Program* (Sacramento: California Legislature Joint Publications, 1987), p. 129.

21. W. Winkelstein, et al., "The San Francisco Men's Health Study: Reduction in Human Immunodeficiency Virus Among Homosexual/Bisexual Men, 1982-84," *American Journal of Public Health* (June, 1987).

22. AIDS Discrimination Unit, "AIDS and People of Color: The Discriminatory Impact" (New York: New York City Commission on Human Rights, Nov. 13, 1986, xerox); "Access of Hispanics to Health Care and Cuts in Services: A State-of-the-Art Overview," *American Journal of Public Health* (May-June, 1986).

23. J. Jackson and L. Rotkiewicz, "A Coupon Program: AIDS Education and Drug Treatment." Paper presented at the Third International Conference on AIDS (Washington, D.C.: June, 1987).

24. J. Mondanaro, "Strategies of AIDS Prevention: Motivating Health Behavior in Drug Dependent Women," *Journal of Psychoactive Drugs*, Vol. 19, No. 2 (April-June, 1987).

25. "Antibody to Human Immunodeficiency Virus in Female Prostitutes," *JAMA*, Vol. 257, No. 15 (April 17, 1987).

26. For a review of these changes, see Sheryl Ruzek, Virginia Olesen and Adele Clark, Women's Health: Complexities and Differences, Columbus: Ohio State University, 1997.

27. In his "Introduction" to *Brother to Brother: New Writings by Black Gay Men*, poet and essayist Essex Hemphill suggests that the notion of "coming home" is more appro-

priate than "coming out" for African American men. "Coming home" refers to one's reintegration as a gay man within the African American community, and throughout its many institutions (Boston: Alyson Publications, 1991).

28. Community organizing projects are complex and their study requires appropriate methodology. One goal of AIDS prevention research in this area should be comparison of the effectiveness of different organizing strategies in controlling the AIDS epidemic. United States research could be done in several African American and Latino communities within one large metropolitan area or state (in order to control for epidemiological and/or political factors). Several organizing techniques could be studied. Interventions could include not only the community organizing per se, but a variety of such AIDS-prevention techniques as support groups, effective use of the media, behavior modification, counseling, and so on.

Data concerning the organizing processes and their impact on the community's institutions and social relations, including individual behavior, should be collected over time. The natural complexity of human social relationships and social change requires the collection and analysis of qualitative as well as quantitative data. And because we know that intervention of any sort is better than nothing in preventing AIDS, it would not be ethical to have a "control" community with no intervention as part of the sample under study, although one could examine epidemiological data from similar communities which did not have intervention and/or research projects.

Index